Current Management of Hepatitis C Virus

Editor

FRED POORDAD

CLINICS IN LIVER DISEASE

www.liver.theclinics.com

Consulting Editor
NORMAN GITLIN

November 2015 • Volume 19 • Number 4

ELSEVIER

1600 John F. Kennedy Boulevard • Suite 1800 • Philadelphia, Pennsylvania, 19103-2899

http://www.theclinics.com

CLINICS IN LIVER DISEASE Volume 19, Number 4
November 2015 ISSN 1089-3261, ISBN-13: 978-0-323-41336-7

Editor: Kerry Holland
Developmental Editor: Meredith Clinton

Clinics in Liver Disease (ISSN 1089-3261) is published quarterly by Elsevier Inc., 360 Park Avenue South, New York, NY 10010-1710. Months of issue are February, May, August, and November. Business and Editorial Offices: 1600 John F. Kennedy Blvd., Ste. 1800, Philadelphia, PA 19103-2899. Customer Service Office: 3251 Riverport Lane, Maryland Heights, MO 63043. Periodicals postage paid at New York, NY and additional mailing offices. Subscription prices are $295.00 per year (U.S. individuals), $145.00 per year (U.S. student/resident), $401.00 per year (U.S. institutions), $395.00 per year (international individuals), $200.00 per year (international student/resident), $498.00 per year (international institutions), $340.00 per year (Canadian individuals), $200.00 per year (Canadian student/resident), and $498.00 per year (Canadian institutions). Foreign air speed delivery is included in all *Clinics* subscription prices. All prices are subject to change without notice. **POSTMASTER:** Send address changes to *Clinics in Liver Disease*, Elsevier Health Sciences Division, Subscription Customer Service, 3251 Riverport Lane, Maryland Heights, MO 63043. **Customer Service: Telephone: 1-800-654-2452 (U.S. and Canada); 314-447-8871 (outside U.S. and Canada). Fax: 314-447-8029. E-mail: journalscustomer service-usa@elsevier.com (for print support); journalsonlinesupport-usa@elsevier.com (for online support).**

Reprints. For copies of 100 or more of articles in this publication, please contact the Commercial Reprints Department, Elsevier Inc., 360 Park Avenue South, New York, NY 10010-1710. Tel.: 212-633-3874; Fax: 212-633-3820; E-mail: reprints@elsevier.com.

Clinics in Liver Disease is covered in *MEDLINE/PubMed (Index Medicus)*, Science Citation Index Expanded, Journal Citation Reports/Science Edition, and Current Contents/Clinical Medicine.

Contributors

CONSULTING EDITOR

NORMAN GITLIN, MD, FRCP (LONDON), FRCPE (EDINBURGH), FAASLD, FACP, FACG
Formerly, Professor of Medicine, Chief of Hepatology, Emory University; Currently,
Consultant, Atlanta Gastroenterology Associates, Atlanta, Georgia

EDITOR

FRED POORDAD, MD
Clinical Professor of Medicine, Chief, Hepatology, University of Texas Health Science
Center at San Antonio; VP, Academic and Clinical Affairs, Texas Liver Institute, San
Antonio, Texas

AUTHORS

WALID S. AYOUB, MD
Assistant Medical Director, Liver Transplant; Associate Professor of Medicine,
Department of Gastroenterology, Cedars Sinai Medical Center, Los Angeles, California

KRISTINA R. CHACKO, MD
Assistant Professor of Medicine, Division of Hepatology, Department of Medicine,
Montefiore Einstein Liver Center, Montefiore Medical Center, Albert Einstein College of
Medicine, Bronx, New York

VANESSA COSTILLA, MD
Department of Hepatology, University of Texas Health Science Center at San Antonio, San
Antonio, Texas

PAUL J. GAGLIO, MD, FACP, AGAF, FAASLD
Medical Director, Adult Liver Transplantation; Professor of Clinical Medicine, Division of
Hepatology, Department of Medicine, Montefiore Einstein Liver Center, Montefiore
Medical Center, Albert Einstein College of Medicine, Bronx, New York

JULIO A. GUTIERREZ, MD, MS
Department of Hepatology, University of Texas Health Science Center at San Antonio; The
Texas Liver Institute, San Antonio, Texas

HOPE HUBBARD, MD
Assistant Professor of Medicine, University of Texas Health Science Center at San
Antonio, San Antonio, Texas

VANDANA KHUNGAR, MD, MSc
Assistant Professor of Medicine, Division of Gastroenterology and Hepatology, University
of Pennsylvania, Philadelphia, Pennsylvania

TATYANA KUSHNER, MD
Gastroenterology Fellow, Division of Gastroenterology and Hepatology, University of Pennsylvania, Philadelphia, Pennsylvania

PAUL Y. KWO, MD
Professor of Medicine, Gastroenterology/Hepatology Division; Medical Director, Liver Transplantation, Indiana University Health, Indiana University School of Medicine, Indianapolis, Indiana

ERIC LAWITZ, MD
Clinical Professor of Medicine, Texas Liver Institute; University of Texas Health Science Center at San Antonio, San Antonio, Texas

NEHA MATHUR, MD
Department of Hepatology, University of Texas Health Science Center at San Antonio, San Antonio, Texas

NANCY REAU, MD
Associate Professor of Medicine, Center for Liver Diseases, University of Chicago Medical Center, Chicago, Illinois

VARUN SAXENA, MD, MS
Division of Gastroenterology and Hepatology, Department of Medicine, University of California, San Francisco, San Francisco, California

ANOUAR TERIAKY, MD, FRCPC
Transplant Hepatology Fellow, Center for Liver Diseases, University of Chicago Medical Center, Chicago, Illinois

NORAH TERRAULT, MD, MPH
Professor of Medicine and Transplant Surgery, Division of Gastroenterology and Hepatology, Department of Medicine, University of California, San Francisco, San Francisco, California

TRAM T. TRAN, MD
Medical Director, Liver Transplant; Associate Professor of Medicine, Cedars Sinai Medical Center, Los Angeles, California

JOHN VIZUETE, MD, MPH
Gastroenterology Fellow, University of Texas Health Science Center at San Antonio, San Antonio, Texas

DAVID L. WYLES, MD
Associate Professor of Medicine, Division of Infectious Diseases, University of California San Diego, La Jolla, California

Contents

Hepatitis C is a major worldwide cause of liver morbidity and mortality. A substantial proportion of infected patients will develop chronic disease, which may progress over decades to cirrhosis. This can lead to decompensation and hepatocellular carcinoma. With the advent of the direct-acting antivirals, hepatitis C has become increasingly curable with limited adverse events and a shorter duration of therapy. This review discusses the evaluation process of the hepatitis C patient in the direct-acting antiviral era, including screening, clinical evaluation, drug-drug interactions, treatment urgency, and counseling.

This article discusses direct-acting antiviral agents that target hepatitis C virus replication, their mechanism of action, strengths, and weaknesses. In addition, varying strategies using combinations of these agents are discussed.

Hepatitis C virus (HCV) infection is a leading cause of cirrhosis and hepatocellular carcinoma, globally. Most individuals infected with HCV are asymptomatic. The introduction of the newer direct-acting antiviral (DAA) therapies has led to achievement of treatment success rates of more than 90%. Sustained virologic response is the end point of therapy, and is considered a virologic cure. It is defined as undetectable HCV RNA 12 weeks after end of therapy. This article reviews current approved non–interferon-based therapy and data from clinical trials in treatment-naive patients with chronic HCV infection.

Over the past few years, tremendous advances have been made in the treatment of hepatitis C with direct-acting antiviral agents (DAAs), allowing treatment options for patients who have failed prior treatment with interferon. In addition to interferon's severe adverse effect profile, and the inability of many patients to tolerate it, prior interferon-containing regimens were not as effective in achieving sustained virologic response as emerging therapies. New DAAs have demonstrated higher rates of sustained virologic response, shorter duration of treatment, and improved adverse effect profile.

The current standard of care for hepatitis C therapy is the combination of direct-acting antiviral (DAA) agents. These orally administered medications target the viral proteins and halt the hepatitis C virus lifecycle. Despite high cure rates with these novel drugs, virologic failure with DAAs are of mounting concern as real-world sustained virologic response 12 rates seem lower than expected. The mechanisms of virologic failure to DAAs are likely multifactorial, including baseline resistance variants, the efficacy of the agents used, and host factors. Salvage therapy for DAA virologic failures is an area of emerging research.

Therapy for hepatitis C has entered the era of all-oral direct-acting antiviral agents. Sustained response rates are now greater than 90% for all genotypes, although patients with cirrhosis remain the most difficult to treat. There are limited data for patients with cirrhosis and with hepatitis C genotypes 4 and 6 with cirrhosis. Genotype 3 patients with cirrhosis need additional strategies to achieve the sustained virologic response rates seen in genotype 1 patients with cirrhosis. This article outlines the currently available therapies for patients with cirrhosis and hepatitis C across all genotypes, with suggested management strategies.

Chronic hepatitis C virus (HCV) infection currently remains the leading indication for liver transplant in the United States. However, recurrent HCV infection after transplant is universal in those who enter transplant with viremia resulting in reduced posttransplant graft and patient survival rates, caused in large part by progressive recurrent HCV disease. Therefore, successful treatment of HCV in the peri-transplant period, either before or after transplant, is paramount in ensuring improved posttransplant outcomes. This article reviews the experience to date treating HCV in waitlisted patients and liver transplant recipients and the unique challenges encountered when treating this population.

Hepatitis C virus (HCV) coinfection is prevalent in patients with human immunodeficiency virus (HIV) and has an accelerated disease course. Direct-acting antiviral (DAA) therapies that do not require interferon increase response rates to levels identical to those seen in HCV monoinfection. However, drug-drug interaction between antiretrovirals and HCV medication is the major consideration in deciding on the appropriate HCV therapeutic approach in patients with HIV. This article summarizes the currently available data with HCV DAAs in patients with HIV, and focuses on predicting and managing drug interaction to facilitate successful DAA-based HCV therapy in those with HIV.

The treatment of chronic hepatitis C virus (HCV) has undergone a period of rapid evolution. The era of combination direct antivirals has led to high rates of sustained viral response (SVR), limited toxicities, and more broad applicability across patient demographics. Even current therapies have their limitations, however, including genotype specificity and variable durations of treatment depending on the presence or absence of cirrhosis. Developing a fixed-duration pangenotypic regimen that can broadly treat all stages of fibrosis with equal rates of SVR in all patients, irrespective of treatment experience, is the goal of future therapies. This article reviews antivirals in development.

CLINICS IN LIVER DISEASE

THE CLINICS ARE AVAILABLE ONLINE!
Access your subscription at:
www.theclinics.com

Preface

Hepatitis C Therapy: Simple for the Patient, not so Simple for the Clinician

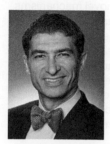

Fred Poordad, MD
Editor

Not since the late 1990s with the arrival of highly active anti-retroviral therapy for HIV has there been such an explosion of new compounds and regimens in the field of virology. The slow beginnings of this new era, the direct-acting antiviral (DAA) therapy for hepatitis C, started a few years ago with the first protease inhibitors, boceprevir and telaprevir, each being paired with interferon and ribavirin, leading to a significant improvement in response rates, but only in the easiest-to-cure population of treatment-naïve patients with genotype 1 virus. For other populations, the poor benefit/risk profile did not justify the widespread use of such toxic regimens.

It was not until all-oral regimens became available that previous predictors of treatment failure were eliminated, including gender, ethnicity, weight, past treatment experience, HIV/HCV coinfection, posttransplantation, and even cirrhosis. So, that made it easier, right? Well, perhaps for the patient and for the clinician managing side effects. However, the field has become more complex for the clinician in terms of understanding mechanisms of how these medications work, the development of resistance, and drug-drug interactions. Unfortunately, one size does not fit all. Different regimens are still required based on genotype and presence, or absence, of cirrhosis, both of which may alter duration.

In this issue of *Clinics in Liver Disease*, Drs Teriaky and Reau discuss how to evaluate the patient with HCV in this modern era, while Drs Chacko and Gaglio review the different classes of DAAs. Drs Ayoub and Tran, and Drs Kushner and Khungar, give overviews of how to treat treatment-naïve and treatment-experienced patients. Drs Costilla, Mathur, and Gutierrez discuss how patients fail these regimens, while Dr Kwo, Drs Saxena and Terrault, and Dr Wyles all summarize the data for special populations such as patients with cirrhosis, peritransplant patients, and HIV/HCV–coinfected patients. Finally, while the hope is that we can eventually cure all

Clin Liver Dis 19 (2015) ix–x
http://dx.doi.org/10.1016/j.cld.2015.08.001
1089-3261/15/$ – see front matter © 2015 Published by Elsevier Inc.

liver.theclinics.com

HCV-infected patients, some patients still fail these highly effective regimens. Drs Vizuete, Hubbard, and Lawitz discuss how best to manage these complicated patients.

Hepatitis C is a curable viral infection and many wonder if it can be eradicated completely someday. While that ambition is a wonderful goal, there is still much work to be done before that. Identifying all patients who are infected, preventing the spread of HCV, and providing access to care/treatment are still major roadblocks for many marginalized individuals.

Importantly, new regimens continue to be developed, and some novel mechanisms of action are being investigated. It will require a few more years, and perhaps other medications, to reach a goal of having an "easy button": one regimen for all patients. That would truly make it simple for clinicians, patients, and the health care system. However, I would not hold my breath. The HCV virus is dynamic, and with the variations we see in the genome, it is very likely that one of several regimens will be chosen based on specific features of the virus and patient. This will then require some evaluation and thought on the part of the clinician to maximize the chances of success for the patient. Simple? No, but it will be effective, and that is all that matters.

Fred Poordad, MD
University of Texas Health Science Center
Texas Liver Institute
607 Camden Street
San Antonio, TX 78215, USA

E-mail address:
poordad@uthscsa.edu

Evaluation of Hepatitis C Patients in the Direct-Acting Antiviral Era

Anouar Teriaky, MD, FRCPC*, Nancy Reau, MD

KEYWORDS

- Hepatitis C • Evaluation • Direct-acting antivirals • Diagnosis • Assessment

KEY POINTS

- Patients at risk for hepatitis C should be screened with hepatitis C virus (HCV) antibody, and active disease should be confirmed by nucleic acid testing, HCV polymerase chain reaction.
- The pretreatment clinical evaluation should consist of a thorough history and physical examination searching for evidence of advanced liver disease or risk factors for progression.
- Initial investigations should include complete blood count, comprehensive metabolic panel, HCV RNA, genotype analysis, HIV, hepatitis A virus and hepatitis B virus serology, and fibrosis staging.
- Numerous drug-drug interactions exist with the direct-acting antivirals, and all medications should be reviewed before initiating treatment.
- Medication adherence is integral to success, and factors that contribute to compliance should be addressed.

INTRODUCTION

The hepatitis C virus (HCV) is a single-stranded RNA enveloped cytoplasmic virus, discovered in 1989.[1] HCV is a major worldwide cause of liver morbidity and mortality. The global prevalence of HCV ranges from 122 to 185 million people or approximately 2.8% of the worldwide population. Areas with the highest prevalence include North Africa, the Middle East, and Central and East Asia.[2] There are 6 genotypes and multiple subtypes. HCV genotypes demonstrate geographic variation and also play an important role in prognosis and therapeutic response.[3]

Dr N. Reau performs consultation work for Abbvie, BMS, and Janssan. Dr N. Reau also receives research support from Abbvie, Gilead, BMS, and Merch. Dr A. Teriaky has nothing to disclose.
Department of Medicine, Center for Liver Diseases, University of Chicago Medical Center, 5841 South Maryland Avenue, Chicago, IL 60637, USA
* Corresponding author.
E-mail address: ateriaky@yahoo.com

Clin Liver Dis 19 (2015) 591–604
http://dx.doi.org/10.1016/j.cld.2015.06.001
1089-3261/15/$ – see front matter © 2015 Elsevier Inc. All rights reserved.

liver.theclinics.com

Eighty percent of HCV-exposed individuals develop chronic disease.[4] The clinical course that follows infection ranges from chronic hepatitis to cirrhosis. Most patients will have a clinically silent course until they develop cirrhosis. Viral and host factors play an important role in the degree and rate of progression of fibrosis.[5–7] The estimated prevalence of cirrhosis after 20 years of chronic HCV infection is approximately 16%.[8] Chronic HCV decreases quality of life, increases liver-related mortality, and increases all-cause mortality.[9,10] Once cirrhotic, the 5-year risk of hepatic decompensation is 18% and hepatocellular carcinoma (HCC) is 7%.[11] After decompensation, the risk of death is 15% to 20% in the following year.[12]

Eradication of HCV can allow regression of fibrosis and cirrhosis in addition to reducing the risk of hepatic decompensation and HCC. Liver-related mortality, all-cause mortality, and quality of life also improve with achieving sustained virologic response (SVR), which is a measure of cure.[13,14] Recent advances in HCV therapy have led to an exciting new era of oral therapies known as the direct-acting antivirals (DAAs). DAAs have minimal adverse events, improved tolerability, and shorter treatment courses and lead to substantially improved SVR. Combined, they offer an all-oral opportunity for cure. This review focuses on the evaluation of HCV patients in the DAA era, including screening, clinical evaluation, drug-drug interactions (DDIs), counseling, and therapeutic considerations.

SCREENING

Identifying chronically infected HCV patients in the population is the first step in the evaluation process. In the United States, 45% to 85% of patients with chronic HCV are unaware of their infection.[15] This finding emphasizes the importance in identifying asymptomatic patients with HCV through screening in order to provide treatment before complications develop. However, random population screening would not be appropriate resource utilization and a more tailored approach is required. Screening should be targeted at individuals with risk factors for HCV infection, evidence of elevated liver enzymes or chronic liver disease of unknown cause, and high prevalence groups. Targeted HCV screening has been shown to be cost-effective in the United States.[16,17] Several organizations in the United States have outlined guidelines for screening for HCV, including the American Association for the Study of Liver Diseases and Centers for Disease Control and Prevention. Although all guidelines agree on the core groups requiring screening, some slight variations do exist.[15,18–22] Appropriate patients should be tested once in a lifetime unless there is ongoing concern for exposure.

Because HCV is a blood-borne infection, risk revolves around blood-mediated mechanisms with active or remote intravenous drug and transfusions before 1992 being important risk factors. Although there has been an association between high-risk sexual behavior and HCV in some studies, others have shown that HCV is inefficiently transmitted sexually possibly showing an association skewed by confounders.[23] Although important, risk factor–based testing misses a substantial proportion of HCV-positive patients when taken alone.[24] Studies have identified a birth cohort between 1945 and 1965 at high risk of HCV. In the National Health and Nutrition Examination Surveys, 81% of the total estimated population with chronic HCV was born between 1945 and 1965.[25] Not all patients had risk factors for HCV. Other HCV risk factors and high prevalence populations are listed in **Box 1**.[15,18–22] Controversial areas for screening include immigrants from high prevalence areas and pregnant women.

Screening for HCV should begin with immunoassays that identify anti-HCV immunoglobulin G (IgG). A positive test should be followed with HCV RNA to confirm active

---

Box 1
Hepatitis C virus screening recommendations in the United States based on hepatitis C virus risk factors and high prevalence populations

Active or remote intravenous drug use

Intranasal drugs

Clotting factors before 1987

Blood products before 1992

Organ transplantation before 1992

Obtaining unregulated tattoos

Being born to an HCV-positive mother

Needlestick or splash injury in a health care worker from an HCV-positive patient

Multiple sexual partners or sex with an intravenous drug user

Birth cohort between 1945 and 1965

Incarcerated patients

Chronic hemodialysis patients

HIV-positive patients

Elevated transaminases or chronic liver disease of unknown cause

Modified from Refs.[15,18–22]

---

infection. Although false positives are rare, they are more common in low-prevalence populations, patients with autoimmune liver disease, and patients with hypergammaglobulinemia. False negatives are also unusual, but can occur in immunocompromised populations such as transplant recipients, HIV patients, and hemodialysis patients.[26] HCV RNA can be performed if suspicion is high. The sensitivity and specificity of third-generation multiantigen immunoassays are 98.9% and 100%.[27,28] These immunoassays can detect anti-HCV IgG as early as 10 weeks after exposure.[29] Rapid assays are also available for point-of-care testing.[30]

CLINICAL EVALUATION

Although many comorbid conditions precluded treatment in the interferon era, the clinical evaluation in the DAA era is now focused on factors that increase risk of progression and impact adherence with few contraindications existing for treatment. The clinical evaluation for patients with HCV begins with a thorough history. Most patients with chronic HCV tend to be asymptomatic unless manifestations of portal hypertension are present. When symptoms occur, they tend to be nonspecific, and severity is not associated with the degree of disease. The most common complaint tends to be fatigue. **Box 2** lists symptoms associated with HCV.[31]

The history should include questions tailored around complications of portal hypertension or decompensation, such as gastrointestinal bleeding, ascites, hepatic encephalopathy, and jaundice. Extrahepatic manifestations can be seen in up to 40% of patients and may regress with therapy.[29] These manifestations should be identified through a combination of history, physical examination, and investigations. The strength of association of these manifestations with HCV is quite variable. **Box 3** lists established extrahepatic manifestations.[29,32]

Box 2
Associated signs and symptoms of patients with hepatitis C virus
Fatigue
Anorexia
Nausea
Abdominal discomfort
Pruritus
Arthralgias
Myalgias
Paresthesias
Difficulty concentrating
Weakness
Weight loss
Adapted from Wright TL, Manns MP. Hepatitis C. In: Boyer TD, Wright TL, Manns MP, editors. Zakim and Boyer's hepatology: a textbook of liver disease. 5th edition. Philadelphia: Elsevier; 2006. p. 670.

Factors that may accelerate progression of liver disease need to be determined from the history. Comorbidities that could influence treatment include cardiovascular disease, which can be exacerbated by anemia with ribavirin regimens, and diabetes, which may increase fibrosis as well as improve with viral eradication. A family history of liver disease should be ruled out. A psychiatric history is still required because an untreated psychiatric illness may require management first to improve compliance. Medication lists should be reviewed for DDIs and potential allergies such as sulfa. A social history with screening for drug and alcohol misuse is necessary to provide appropriate counseling and support.

The physical examination should revolve around assessing for evidence of chronic liver disease. Stigmata of chronic liver disease that may be seen in HCV includes palmar erythema, clubbing, muscle wasting, fetor hepaticus, spider angiomata, gynecomastia, feminization of body hair, caput medusa, testicular atrophy, scleral icterus, and jaundice. Abdominal examination should assess for liver nodularity, splenomegaly, and ascites. Overt hepatic encephalopathy can be diagnosed through neurologic assessment for asterixis and a mental status evaluation.

Pretreatment Investigations

The purpose of pretreatment investigations is to confirm the diagnosis, to rule out other causes of liver disease and comorbidities that may impact treatment, to stage the disease, and to identify extrahepatic manifestations if present.

Hepatitis C Virus Investigations

If anti-HCV IgG is positive on screening, HCV RNA should follow it. HCV RNA is the gold standard for diagnosis of active HCV and can be seen in serum as soon as 1 week after infection.[30] The viral load impacts SVR and duration of therapy, but not virulence. HCV RNA tests are both quantitative and qualitative. These nucleic acid tests for detecting HCV RNA are based on polymerase chain reaction, transcription-mediated amplification, and branched DNA testing technology. The World Health

---

Box 3
Extrahepatic manifestations of hepatitis C virus

Dermatologic

Porphyria cutanea tarda

Lichen planus

Cutaneous vasculitis

Purpura

Vitiligo

Endocrine

Autoimmune thyroiditis

Thyroid cancer

Diabetes mellitus

Hematologic

Mixed cryoglobulinemia

Non-Hodgkin lymphoma

Monoclonal gammopathies

Renal

Membranoproliferative glomerulonephritis

Membranous nephropathy

Renal cell carcinoma

Rheumatologic

Raynaud's

Chronic polyarthritis

Sicca syndrome

Respiratory

Idiopathic pulmonary fibrosis

Neurologic

Sensory neuropathy

Motor neuropathy

Adapted from Cacoub P, Renou C, Rosenthal E, et al. Extrahepatic manifestations associated with hepatitis C virus infection. A prospective multicenter study of 321 patients. The GERMIVIC. Groupe d'Etude et de Recherche en Medecine Interne et Maladies Infectieuses sur le Virus de l'Hepatite C. Medicine 2000;79:49; and O'Leary JG, Davis GL. Hepatitis C. In: Feldman M, Friedman LS, Brandt LJ, editors. Sleisenger and Fordtran's: gastrointestinal and liver disease. 9th edition. Philadelphia: Elsevier; 2010. p. 1320.

Organization standardized all HCV RNA detection, which is now expressed in international units (IU) to minimize variability.[33] Quantitative tests quantitate HCV RNA and have become extremely sensitive, detecting as little as 5 IU/mL.[34] A baseline viral load is essential before initiating therapy. With the high sensitivity of quantitative methods, utilization of qualitative methods is likely to decline. Qualitative methods can detect very low levels of HCV RNA, which can confirm the diagnosis as well as SVR after treatment.

HCV genotype analysis is essential before treatment because it impacts the duration of therapy and treatment regimen used and prognosticates outcomes. Genotype 3 is the most virulent leading to an increased risk of cirrhosis and HCC and seems to be the most difficult to eradicate with the currently available DAAs.[35,36]

Other Investigations

Initial blood work should include a complete blood count (CBC) with careful attention to the hemoglobin for evidence of anemia, which could impact treatment choices especially with ribavirin regimens. The platelet count should also be reviewed for thrombocytopenia, which may indicate portal hypertension.[37] A comprehensive metabolic panel (CMP) should be assessed for evidence of elevated transaminases or synthetic liver dysfunction. Transaminases do not always correlate with the degree of necroinflammation and may be normal despite advanced fibrosis.[38] Renal function is assessed by the creatinine and glomerular filtration rate, which are included in the CMP.[39] Creatinine can be an unreliable measure of renal function in patients with cirrhosis due to muscle wasting. Patients with end-stage renal disease presently have limited options with the available DAA therapies. The international normalized ratio (INR) can offer additional measure of synthetic liver function.

Routine testing for DAA resistance mutations has not been advocated historically,[39] but may become a part of the initial and ongoing assessment around treatment. The presence of baseline variants will require selection of regimens that do not have liabilities to that variant. Currently, testing is available for both the NS3 region of the virus and the NS5A region.

In female patients of child-bearing age, a negative pregnancy test should be established. Patients must be taking appropriate contraception especially when starting a ribavirin regimen, because ribavirin is potentially harmful to the fetus. Patients and partners must avoid pregnancy for at least 6 months after ribavirin exposure.[39] Testing for coinfection with hepatitis B and HIV due to the common route of transmission is necessary. Assessing for hepatitis A immunity is also recommended. If not immune to hepatitis A and B, patients should be counseled regarding vaccination to prevent further hepatic deterioration.[39] If there is a concern for ongoing substance abuse, a toxicology screen may be appropriate as well as appropriate counseling and linkage to support networks to achieve abstinence.

Other causes of liver disease should be excluded (**Box 4**). If there is concern for extrahepatic manifestation of HCV on clinical assessment, further investigations should be considered. For example, if there is suspicion for cryoglobulinemia, cryoglobulins, complement levels, and rheumatoid factor should be ordered. Imaging has generally been performed on initial presentation to assess for steatosis, hepatosplenomegaly, hepatic masses, and ascites. If cirrhotic, the extent of liver dysfunction should be determined by calculation of the Model of End-stage Liver Disease score. If a patient's score is 15 or greater, they should be managed by an experienced provider, which could include referral to a liver transplant center.[40]

HCV patients that have evidence of cirrhosis require appropriate surveillance for varices and HCC. A screening esophagogastroduodenoscopy should be performed at the time of diagnosis with cirrhosis, and follow-up procedures will be dependent on the findings. HCC screening is also required at 6-month intervals with ultrasound in these patients. If HCV is eradicated, patients with cirrhosis still require regular screening. Hepatic encephalopathy and ascites should be managed in a similar fashion to other cirrhotic patients. Some of the DAAs have been studied in decompensated cirrhosis, whereas interferon is contraindicated in this population.

Box 4
Initial investigations before treatment in hepatitis C virus patients

CBC

CMP

INR

HCV genotype analysis

Quantitative HCV RNA

Anti-HAV (total or IgG)

HBsAg, anti-HBc, anti-HBs

HIV

Toxicology screen (as necessary)

Pregnancy testing

Abdominal ultrasound

Screening for other causes chronic liver disease (as necessary): ANA, ASMA, AMA, immunoglobulins, ceruloplasmin, α1 antitrypsin phenotype, ferritin, transferrin saturation

Fibrosis staging

Abbreviations: AMA, antimitochondrial antibody; ANA, antinuclear antibody; anti-HAV, hepatitis A virus antibody; anti-HBc, hepatitis B core antibody; anti-HBs, hepatitis B surface antibody; ASMA, antismooth muscle antibody; HBsAg, hepatitis B surface antigen.

Fibrosis Staging

Fibrosis staging is the single most impactful factor in the evaluation process. The degree of fibrosis drives the urgency for therapy and has implications regarding duration of therapy and treatment efficacy and holds important prognostic value in determining the risk of morbidity and mortality. Cirrhotic patients also require regular assessment, including HCC screening, to prevent complications.[41]

Staging methods can be divided into noninvasive and invasive. Noninvasive methods are further divided into radiologic and serologic tests. Radiologic tests include conventional imaging and novel elastography techniques. Serologic tests can be separated into numerous indirect and direct markers of fibrosis. Invasive methods include percutaneous and transjugular liver biopsies. The noninvasive methods have led to a reduced need for liver biopsies in staging the extent of HCV, but not all techniques have widespread availability.

Conventional radiologic imaging includes ultrasound, computed tomography, and MRI. These methods provide complementary information supporting cirrhosis, but cannot be interpreted alone. They do not reliably differentiate the various stages of fibrosis. Features on cross-sectional imaging seen with cirrhosis include parenchymal nodularity and heterogeneity, segmental lobe hypertrophy and atrophy, and features of portal hypertension.[42,43]

Elastography is a novel noninvasive imaging technique that allows liver stiffness to be determined by mapping the elastic properties of soft tissue. Most elastography methods can differentiate minimal fibrosis from significant fibrosis, but cannot reliably differentiate the stages of fibrosis. Transient elastography (Fibroscan) uses 1-dimensional ultrasound to determine liver stiffness based on shear wave propagation. Results are represented in kilopascals (kPa) with the cutoffs for a diagnosis of significant fibrosis (METAVIR F $\geq$2) and cirrhosis, respectively, greater than 7 and greater than

12.5 kPa.[44] Magnetic resonance elastography involves combining MRI technology with vibrations emitted through a transducer, which produces a shear elasticity map of the entire liver. Other elastography techniques include acoustic radiation force imaging and real-time shear wave elastography. These techniques combine conventional ultrasound with elastography. All these methods perform well when differentiating minimal fibrosis from cirrhosis.[45–48] Comparing these different methods of elastography is beyond the scope of this review because they all have inherent strengths and weaknesses.

Serologic markers of fibrosis are divided into indirect and direct markers. Indirect markers exhibit changes of hepatic function, whereas direct markers signify extracellular matrix turnover, which is directly influenced by hepatic fibrosis.[43] There are several markers that have been studied, and the most widely available are focused on and are listed in **Table 1**. Serologic markers can also differentiate mild fibrosis from cirrhosis, but cannot reliably differentiate intermediate stages of fibrosis. Most serologic markers are useful in identifying significant fibrosis or cirrhosis.[49] Some serologic markers such as the aspartate aminotransferase (AST) to platelet ratio index (APRI) and FIB-4 (Fibrosis-4) can be calculated from basic blood work, while others require patented formulas consisting of biochemical and clinical markers, which are expressed as a numerical value that correlates with the degree of fibrosis.[49–54] Combining various noninvasive radiologic and serologic methods to assess for significant fibrosis has been shown to improve fibrosis assessment and minimize the need for invasive testing.[55,56]

Invasive methods for fibrosis staging have long been the gold standard, but they can be an imperfect test. Biopsies can be poorly representative of the whole liver if a limited sample size is obtained. Patients are at risk of complications with the potential for significant adverse events. One benefit of a biopsy is the ability to also determine the degree of inflammation, which has prognostic value, and diagnose concomitant liver diseases such as steatosis. With the advent of noninvasive tests, fewer liver biopsies are being performed.[43]

Table 1
Various serologic tests to assess for significant fibrosis/cirrhosis in hepatitis C virus patients

Serologic Test	Components	Cutoff
Platelet count	Platelets	<150,000 μ/L
APRI	(AST/ULN AST)/platelets × 100	>1.0
Fibrosure or fibrotest	α-2-Macroglobulin, GGT, apolipoprotein A1, haptoglobin, total bilirubin, age, gender	>0.8
Hepascore	Bilirubin, GGT, hyaluronic acid, α-2-macroglobulin, age, gender	≥0.55
Fibroindex	Platelets, AST, γ-globulin	≥2.25
FIB-4	Platelets, AST, ALT, age	>3.25
Forns index	Age, GGT, cholesterol, platelets	>6.9
Fibrometer	Platelets, PT, AST, α-2-macroglobulin, hyaluronic acid, BUN, age	>0.59
Fibrospect II	Hyaluronic acid, TIMP-1, α-2-macroglobulin	≥0.42
Enhanced liver fibrosis panel	Hyaluronic acid level, aminoterminal propeptide of type III collagen level, TIMP-1, age	≥9.8

Abbreviations: ALT, alanine aminotransferase; AST, aspartate aminotransferase; BUN, blood urea nitrogen; FIB-4, fibrosis-4; GGT, gamma-glutamyl transferase; TIMP-1, tissue inhibitor of metalloproteinase-1; ULN, upper limit of normal.
Data from Refs.[49–54]

DRUG-DRUG INTERACTIONS

With the advent of the DAA era, there has been an improvement in SVR. However, the numerous DAAs for treating HCV still have DDIs that need to be carefully reviewed before initiating therapy. DDIs can lead to a change in drug concentration or cause an additive or opposing effect without altering the concentration by inducing or inhibiting pathways. Many DAAs are metabolized by the cytochrome P450 (CYP) 3A pathway or transported by the P-glycoprotein (P-gp). Thus, they can exert an inhibitory effect on CYP3A and P-gp, which can alter drug metabolism. Other CYP pathways, enzymes, and transporters may also be involved.[57]

Table 2 lists drugs that should not be coadministered with DAAs and ribavirin because of significant DDIs.[58] Other potential drug interactions exist that require intensified monitoring, a change in dosage, or adjustment in administration. For example, potential interactions with ledipasvir/sofosbuvir include specific antiarrhythmics, HIV antiretrovirals, and some statin agents. Acid-reducing agents, such as proton pump inhibitors, should be reviewed because they can decrease drug absorption and lead to lower antiviral efficacy. With the combination of ombitasvir/paritaprevir/ritonavir/dasabuvir, potential interactions also include specific antiarrhythmics, antifungals, calcium channel blockers, HIV antiretrovirals, inhalers, immunosuppresants, statins, diuretics, proton pump inhibitors, analgesics, and sedatives. For a detailed and up-to-date guide on specific DDIs, refer to http://www.hep-druginteractions. org.[58] Most drugs with potential interactions can be modified and do not preclude treatment.

COUNSELING

Patients should be educated on transmission, prognosis, and the natural history of HCV and what evaluation and treatment entail. They should be counseled on abstaining from behavior that can expedite disease progression such as alcohol abuse. Support should be provided if seeking treatment for substance abuse. Patients should be informed that HCV is not transmitted through household contact. They should also be informed that the risk of sexual transmission in a monogamous relationship is low, and safe sexual practice should be followed. Patients should not share toothbrushes or razors, and they are not candidates for blood donation. They should be provided with local resources such as support groups and online resources on HCV to better educate themselves.[39] Patients should also be counseled regarding reinfection.

WHEN TO TREAT

Ideally all patients with HCV should be treated, because SVR decreases liver-related morbidity and mortality, decreases all-cause mortality, and improves quality of life.[14] DAAs are well tolerated with minimal adverse events, high SVR rates, and short treatment durations. Patients with advanced fibrosis are most likely to immediately benefit from treatment and may possibly reverse fibrosis if successfully treated. The DAAs have been shown to be highly effective even in cirrhotics and special populations such as coinfected patients.[39] Potential barriers to treating all patients with HCV include limited resources, both monetary and health care provider work force. Prioritizing patients by urgency is controversial but common when treating HCV, starting with patients with advanced fibrosis and extrahepatic manifestations. However, if the capacity to treat all patients exists, prioritization is not appropriate.

Table 2
Direct-acting antivirals, ribavirin, and drugs that should not be coadministered because of significant drug-to-drug interactions

HCV Drug	Drugs		
DCV	Carbamazepine	Phenobarbital	Rifampicin
	Dexamethasone	Phenytoin	Rifapentine
	Eslicarbazepine	Rifabutin	St John's wort
	Oxcarbazepine		
LED/SOF	Carbamazepine	Rifabutin	St John's wort
	Oxcarbazepine	Rifampicin	Tipranavir
	Phenobarbital	Rifapentine	
	Phenytoin	Rosuvastatin	
OPRD	Alfuzosin	Ethinylestradiol	Phenobarbital
	Aliskiren	Etravirine	Phenytoin
	Astemizole	Gemfibrozil	Ranolazine
	Bosentan	Halofantrine	Rifampicin
	Carbamazepine	Imatinib	Ritonavir
	Cisapride	Ivabradine	Salmeterol
	Dextropropoxyphene	Lercandipine	Sildenafil
	Dihydroergotamine	Lovastatin	Simvastatin
	Efavirenz	Lumefantrine	St John's wort
	Elvitegravir/cobicistat	Methylergonovine	Sunitinib
	Ergonovine	Midazolam (oral)	Terfenadine
	Ergotamine	Oxcarbazepine	Tipranavir
	Eslicarbazepine	Pimozide	Triazolam
SMV	Atazanavir	Eslicarbazepine	Posaconazole
	Astemizole	Etravirine	Rifabutin
	Carbamazepine	Fluconazole	Rifampicin
	Clarithromycin	Fosamprenavir	Rifapentine
	Cisapride	Indinavir	Ritonavir
	Cyclosporine	Itraconazole	Saquinavir
	Darunavir	Ketoconazole	Silybum
	Delaviridine	Lopinavir	St John's wort
	Dexamethasone	Methylergonovine	Telithromycin
	Dextropropoxyphene	Nelfinavir	Terfenadine
	Dihydroergotamine	Nevirapine	Thioridazine
	Efavirenz	Oxcarbazepine	Tipranavir
	Elvitegravir/cobicistat	Phenobarbital	Troleandomycin
	Ergonovine	Phenytoin	Voriconazole
	Ergotamine	Pimozide	Ziprasidone
	Erythromycin		
SOF	Carbamazepine	Phenytoin	St John's wort
	Oxcarbazepine	Rifabutin	Tipranavir
	Nelfinavir	Rifampicin	
	Phenobarbital	Rifapentine	
RBV	Didanosine	Zidovudine	—

Abbreviations: DCV, daclatasvir; LED/SOF, ledipasvir/sofosbuvir; OPRD, ombitasvir/paritaprevir/ritonavir/dasabuvir; RBV, ribavirin; SMV, simeprevir; SOF, sofosbuvir.

Modified from The hepatitis drug interactions Web site. The University of Liverpool. 2015. Available at: http://www.hep-druginteractions.org. Accessed January 18, 2015.

SUMMARY

In summary, HCV is a major global health problem, which can be better managed with the currently approved all-oral DAAs. The first step in the evaluation process should begin with identifying infected individuals, because HCV remains silent until its later stages. Patients that have chronic HCV should undergo a clinical evaluation to assess the degree of fibrosis and for evidence of extrahepatic manifestations. Initial investigations should include a CBC, CMP, INR, HCV RNA, genotype, HIV, hepatitis A virus and hepatitis B virus serology, and fibrosis staging. All patients should be considered for therapy with patients with advanced fibrosis most likely to benefit. Patients should be screened for DDIs before initiating therapy. Appropriate counseling and resources should be offered to all patients.

REFERENCES

1. Choo QL, Kuo G, Weiner AJ, et al. Isolation of a cDNA clone derived from a blood-borne non-A, non-B viral hepatitis genome. Science 1989;244:359–62.
2. Mohd Hanafiah K, Groeger J, Flaxman AD, et al. Global epidemiology of hepatitis C virus infection: new estimates of age-specific antibody to HCV seroprevalence. Hepatology 2013;57:1333–42.
3. Simmonds P, Bukh J, Combet C, et al. Consensus proposals for a unified system of nomenclature of hepatitis C virus genotypes. Hepatology 2005;42:962–73.
4. Barrera JM, Bruguera M, Ercilla MG, et al. Persistent hepatitis C viremia after acute self-limiting posttransfusion hepatitis C. Hepatology 1995;21:639–44.
5. Grebely J, Page K, Sacks-Davis R, et al. The effect of female sex, viral genotype, and IL28B genotype on spontaneous clearance of acute hepatitis C virus infection. Hepatology 2014;59:109–20.
6. Poynard T, Bedossa P, Opolon P. Natural history of liver fibrosis progression in patients with chronic hepatitis C: the OBSVIRC, METAVIR, CLINIVIR, and DOSVIRC groups. Lancet 1997;349:825–32.
7. Everhart JE, Lok AS, Kim HY, et al. Weight-related effects on disease progression in the hepatitis C antiviral long-term treatment against cirrhosis trial. Gastroenterology 2009;137:549–57.
8. Thien HH, Yi Q, Dore GJ, et al. Estimation of stage-specific fibrosis progression rates in chronic hepatitis C virus infection: a meta-analysis and meta-regression. Hepatology 2008;48:418–31.
9. Spiegel BM, Younossi ZM, Hays RD, et al. Impact of hepatitis C on health related quality of life: a systematic review and quantitative assessment. Hepatology 2005;41:790–800.
10. Lee MH, Yang HI, Lu SN, et al. Chronic hepatitis C virus infection increases mortality from hepatic and extrahepatic diseases: a community-based long-term prospective study. J Infect Dis 2012;206:469–77.
11. Fattovich G, Giustina G, Degos F, et al. Morbidity and mortality in compensated cirrhosis type C: a retrospective follow-up study of 384 patients. Gastroenterology 1997;112:463–72.
12. Westbrook RH, Dushieko J. Natural history of hepatitis C. J Hepatol 2014;61: S58–68.
13. Ng V, Saab S. Effects of a sustained virologic response on outcomes of patients with chronic hepatitis C. Clin Gastroenterol Hepatol 2011;9:923–30.
14. van der Meer AJ, Veldt BJ, Feld JJ, et al. Association between sustained virological response and all-cause mortality among patients with chronic hepatitis C and advanced hepatic fibrosis. JAMA 2012;308:2584–93.

15. Smith BD, Morgan RL, Beckett GA, et al. Recommendations for the identification of chronic hepatitis C virus infection among persons born during 1945-1965. MMWR Recomm Rep 2012;61:1–32.
16. Rein DB, Smith BD, Wittenborn JS, et al. The cost-effectiveness of birth-cohort screening for hepatitis C antibody in U.S. primary care settings. Ann Intern Med 2012;156:263–70.
17. Eckman MH, Talal AH, Gordon SC, et al. Cost-effectiveness of screening for chronic hepatitis C infection in the United States. Clin Infect Dis 2013;56: 1382–93.
18. Ghany MG, Strader DB, Thomas DL, et al. Diagnosis, management, and treatment of hepatitis C: an update. Hepatology 2009;49:1335–74.
19. Workowski KA, Berman S, Centers for Disease Control and Prevention (CDC). Sexually transmitted diseases treatment guidelines, 2010. MMWR Recomm Rep 2010;59:1–110.
20. National Institutes of Health. Management of hepatitis C: 2002. National Institutes of Health. 2002. Available at: http://consensus.nih.gov/2002/2002Hepatitis C2002116html.htm. Accessed January 8, 2015.
21. Moyer VA, U.S. Preventive Services Task Force. Screening for hepatitis C virus infection in adults: U.S. Preventive Services Task Force recommendation statement. Ann Intern Med 2013;159:349–57.
22. Murphy EL, Bryzman SM, Glynn SA, et al. Risk factors for hepatitis C virus infection in United States blood donors. Hepatology 2000;31:756–62.
23. Vandelli C, Renzo F, Romano L, et al. Lack of evidence of sexual transmission of hepatitis C among monogamous couples: results of a 10-year prospective follow up study. Am J Gastroenterol 2004;99:855–9.
24. Chou R, Cottrell EB, Wasson N, et al. Screening for hepatitis C virus infection in adults: a systematic review for the U.S. Preventive Services Task Force. Ann Intern Med 2013;158:101–8.
25. Denniston MM, Jiles RB, Drobeniuc J, et al. Chronic hepatitis C infection in the United States, National Health and Nutrition Examination Survey 2003 to 2010. Ann Intern Med 2014;160:293–300.
26. Albeldawi M, Ruiz-Rodriguez E, Carey WD. Hepatitis C virus: prevention, screening, and interpretation of assays. Cleve Clin J Med 2010;77:616–26.
27. Barrera JM, Francis B, Ercilla G, et al. Improved detection of anti-HCV in post-transfusion hepatitis by a third-generation ELISA. Vox Sang 1995;68:15–8.
28. Colin C, Lanoir D, Touzet S, et al. Sensitivity and specificity of third-generation hepatitis C virus antibody detection assays: an analysis of the literature. J Viral Hepat 2001;8:87–95.
29. Cacoub P, Renou C, Rosenthal E, et al. Extrahepatic manifestations associated with hepatitis C virus infection. A prospective multicenter study of 321 patients. The GERMIVIC. Groupe d'Etude et de Recherche en Medecine Interne et Maladies Infectieuses sur le Virus de l'Hepatite C. Medicine 2000;79:47–56.
30. Shivkumar S, Peeling R, Jafari Y, et al. Accuracy of rapid and point-of-care screening tests for hepatitis C: a systematic review and meta-analysis. Ann Intern Med 2012;157:558–66.
31. Wright TL, Manns MP. Hepatitis C. In: Boyer TD, Wright TL, Manns MP, editors. Zakim and Boyer's hepatology: a textbook of liver disease. 5th edition. Philadelphia: Elsevier; 2006. p. 665–86.
32. O'Leary JG, Davis GL. Hepatitis C. In: Feldman M, Friedman LS, Brandt LJ, editors. Sleisenger and Fordtran's: gastrointestinal and liver disease. 9th edition. Philadelphia: Elsevier; 2010. p. 1313–35.

33. Saldanha J, Heath A, Aberham C, et al. World Health Organization collaborative study to establish a replacement WHO international standard for hepatitis C virus RNA nucleic amplification technology assays. Vox Sang 2005;88:202–4.
34. Pawlotsky JM. Use and interpretation of hepatitis C virus diagnostic assays. Clin Liver Dis 2003;7:127–37.
35. Kanwal F, Kramer JR, Ilyas J, et al. HCV genotype 3 is associated with an increased risk of cirrhosis and hepatocellular cancer in a national sample of U.S. veterans with HCV. Hepatology 2014;60:98–105.
36. Schinazi R, Halfton P, Marcellin P, et al. HCV direct-acting antiviral agents: the best interferon-free combinations. Liver Int 2014;34(Suppl 1):69–78.
37. Lu SN, Wang JH, Liu SL, et al. Thrombocytopenia as a surrogate for cirrhosis and a marker for the identification of patients at high-risk for hepatocellular carcinoma. Cancer 2006;107:2212–22.
38. McCormick SE, Goodman ZD, Maydonovitch CL, et al. Evaluation of liver histology, ALT elevation, and HCV RNA titer in patients with chronic hepatitis C. Am J Gastroenterol 1996;91:1516–22.
39. AASLD/IDSA/IAS–USA. Recommendations for testing, managing, and treating hepatitis C. 2015. Available at: http://www.hcvguidelines.org. Accessed January 14, 2015.
40. Martin P, DiMartini A, Feng S, et al. Evaluation for liver transplantation in adults: 2013 practice guideline by the American Association for the Study of Liver Diseases and the American Society of Transplantation. Hepatology 2014;59: 1144–65.
41. Castera L. Noninvasive methods to assess liver disease in patients with hepatitis B or C. Gastroenterology 2012;142:1293–302.
42. Kudo M, Zheng RQ, Kim SR, et al. Diagnostic accuracy of imaging for liver cirrhosis compared to histologically proven liver cirrhosis. A multicenter collaborative study. Intervirology 2008;51(Suppl 1):17–26.
43. Sharma S, Khalili K, Nguyen GC. Non-invasive diagnosis of advance fibrosis and cirrhosis. World J Gastroenterol 2014;20:16820–30.
44. Castera L, Vergniol J, Foucher J, et al. Prospective comparison of transient elastography, Fibrotest, APRI, and liver biopsy for the assessment of fibrosis in chronic hepatitis C. Gastroenterology 2005;128:343–50.
45. Tsochatzis EA, Gurusamy KS, Ntaoula S, et al. Elastography for the diagnosis of severity of fibrosis in chronic liver disease: a meta-analysis of diagnostic accuracy. J Hepatol 2011;54:650–9.
46. Wang QB, Zhu H, Liu HL, et al. Performance of magnetic resonance elastography and diffusion-weighted imaging for the staging of hepatic fibrosis: a meta-analysis. Hepatology 2012;56:239–47.
47. Crespo G, Fernandez-Varo G, Marino Z, et al. ARFI, FibroScan, ELF, and their combinations in the assessment of liver fibrosis: a prospective study. J Hepatol 2012;57:281–7.
48. Ferraioli G, Tinelli C, Dal Bello B, et al. Accuracy of real-time shear wave elastography for assessing liver fibrosis in chronic hepatitis C: a pilot study. Hepatology 2012;56(6):2125–33.
49. Chou R, Wasson N. Blood tests to diagnose fibrosis or cirrhosis in patients with chronic hepatitis C virus infection: a systematic review. Ann Intern Med 2013; 158:807–20.
50. Lin ZH, Xin YN, Dong QJ, et al. Performance of the aspartate aminotransferase-to-platelet ratio index for the staging of hepatitis C-related fibrosis: an updated meta-analysis. Hepatology 2011;53:726–36.

51. Vallet-Pichard A, Mallet V, Nalpas B, et al. FIB-4: an inexpensive and accurate marker of fibrosis in HCV infection. Comparison with liver biopsy and fibrotest. Hepatology 2007;46:32–6.

52. Halfon P, Bacq Y, De Muret A, et al. Comparison of test performance profile for blood tests of liver fibrosis in chronic hepatitis C. J Hepatol 2007;46:395–402.

53. Patel K, Nelson DR, Rockey DC, et al. Correlation of FIBROSpect II with histologic and morphometric evaluation of liver fibrosis in chronic hepatitis C. Clin Gastroenterol Hepatol 2008;6:242–7.

54. Parker J, Guha IN, Roderick P, et al. Enhanced Liver Fibrosis (ELF) test accurately identifies liver fibrosis in patients with chronic hepatitis C. J Viral Hepat 2011;18: 23–31.

55. Sebastiani G, Vario A, Guido M, et al. Stepwise combination algorithms of non-invasive markers to diagnose significant fibrosis in chronic hepatitis C. J Hepatol 2006;44:686–93.

56. Sebastiani G, Halfon P, Castera L, et al. SAFE biopsy: a validated method for large-scale staging of liver fibrosis in chronic hepatitis C. Hepatology 2009;49: 1821–7.

57. Back D, Else L. The importance of drug-drug interactions in the DAA era. Dig Liver Dis 2013;45(Suppl 5):S343–8.

58. The hepatitis drug interactions website. The University of Liverpool. 2015. Available at: http://www.hep-druginteractions.org. Accessed January 8, 2015.

Meet the Classes of Directly Acting Antiviral Agents: Strengths and Weaknesses

Kristina R. Chacko, MD, Paul J. Gaglio, MD*

KEYWORDS

- Direct-acting antiviral agents • Protease inhibitors • Polymerase inhibitors
- NS5A inhibitors

KEY POINTS

- Understanding the life cycle of hepatitis C virus (HCV) provides the opportunity to directly target and inhibit key components required for viral replication.
- Combining direct-acting antiviral therapies can successfully eradicate HCV by inhibiting viral replication.
- Different classes of direct-acting antiviral agents have different potency, barriers to resistance, and toxicities.

INTRODUCTION

Infection with hepatitis C virus (HCV) contributes to substantial worldwide morbidity and mortality. Chronic liver injury induced by the virus may produce hepatocellular injury and fibrosis with progression to cirrhosis, leading to significant consequences including portal hypertension, liver cancer, and death. Cirrhosis caused by HCV represents the most common indication for liver transplantation in the United States, and one of the most common causes of liver cancer worldwide. Over the last few years, efficacy and tolerability of HCV therapy have improved dramatically, and all-oral direct-acting antiviral (DAA) therapies that effectively inhibit viral replication are now available. This article discusses the various classes of DAAs, outlines their strengths and weaknesses, and discusses strategies to combine these agents to achieve optimal results.

Dr P.J. Gaglio has received research support from Abbvie, BMS, BI, Gilead, Merck, Janssen, and has served on advisory boards for Abbvie, BMS, BI, Gilead, Merck and Janssen. Dr K.R. Chacko has nothing to disclose.
Division of Hepatology, Department of Medicine, Montefiore Einstein Liver Center, Montefiore Medical Center, Albert Einstein College of Medicine, 111 East 210 Street Rosenthal 2 Red Zone, Bronx, NY 10467, USA
* Corresponding author.
E-mail address: pgaglio@montefiore.org

THE HEPATITIS C VIRUS LIFE CYCLE

Understanding the HCV life cycle has facilitated the development of novel, targeted DAAs that effectively inhibit viral replication. HCV was originally identified in 1989 as a single-stranded, positive sense RNA virus. It consists of the RNA genome, core protein, and envelope glycoproteins E1 and E2. The HCV particle has a viral envelope consisting of low-density lipoprotein (LDL) and very low-density lipoprotein (VLDL) that anchors the envelope glycoproteins.[1] Therefore, it is has been observed that hepatocellular lipid metabolism and lipid receptors play an important role in the HCV life cycle. Apolipoproteins, especially apolipoprotein E (ApoE), are highly associated with HCV particles and are involved both in viral entry into the hepatocyte and viral replication.[2]

VIRAL ENTRY

HCV attaches to the hepatocyte cell surface through interactions with scavenger receptor B1 (SRB1) and heparan sulfate proteoglycan syndecan-1.[3] The viral particle gains entry into hepatocytes through a complex process involving viral envelope glycoproteins and host cellular molecules. Cell surface protein CD81 is a tetraspanin protein located on hepatocytes and other cell types whose extracellular loop binds HCV E2 and mediates internalization of the virus into the hepatocyte, with claudin-1 (CLDN-1) serving as a vital co-factor.[4] SRB1 also plays a significant role in viral entry, both through interactions with the lipid-rich viral particle and direct binding of E2.[5] Additional host cell surface molecules, including glycosaminoglycans, members of the claudin family (CLDN1, 6 and 9), occludin, epidermal growth factor receptor, and mannose-binding lectins DC-SIGN and L-SIGN serve as receptors or coreceptors and are involved in HCV binding and entry.[6] The association of HCV with lipoproteins suggests an important role for the LDL receptor in the HCV life cycle. Although originally thought to be involved in viral entry, it appears that the LDL receptor is linked to postentry viral replication[7] (**Fig. 1**).[8]

VIRAL REPLICATION

After undergoing fusion and uncoating, the RNA virus is translated into a unique polyprotein mediated by the internal ribosome entry site (IRES).[8] During post-translational processing, the HCV polyprotein subsequently undergoes cleavage by host and viral peptidases into structural proteins (core protein C, envelope glycoproteins E1 and E2, p7) and nonstructural proteins (NS2, NS3, NS4A, NS4B, NS5A, and NS5B). NS2, a zinc-dependent metalloproteinase, is a viral peptidase that cleaves NS2 from NS3. NS3 assembles with its cofactor, NS4A, creating NS3/4A protease, which cleaves the downstream NS proteins, NS4A-NS4B, NS4B-NS5A, and NS5A-NS5B (**Fig. 2**[8] and **Fig. 3**[9]).

Together, the various NS proteins are responsible for HCV replication. NS4B functions as a scaffold, inducing rearrangements of intracytoplasmic membranes into a membranous web that serves as the HCV replication complex.[3] All NS proteins, as well as a number of host factors, play important roles in the creation of the membranous web, leading to HCV replication. NS5A is a zinc–metalloprotein involved in assembly and regulation of the replication complex, and it interacts with host enzymes cyclophilin A and phosphatidylinositol 4-kinase IIIa (PI4KIIIa) to serve as a modulator of the life cycle of the virus.[10] Cyclophilin A, a vital HCV replication factor, aids in protein folding and regulates polyprotein processing. PI4KIIIa is a lipid kinase residing in the endoplasmic reticulum (ER) membrane responsible for the phosphorylation of NS5A.[11] NS5B, an RNA-dependent RNA polymerase (RdRp), is the key enzyme controlling RNA synthesis.

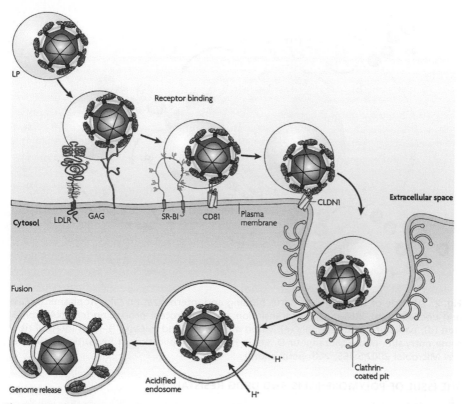

Fig. 1. HCV binding to hepatocyte. CLDN-1, claudin 1; GAG, glycosaminoglycans; LDLR, low density lipoprotein receptor; LP, very low density lipoproteins; SR-B1, scavenger receptor class B type. (*From* Moradpour D, Penin F, Rice C. Replication of hepatitis C virus. Nat Rev Microbiol 2007;5:456; with permission.)

Structural proteins are involved in viral assembly and release with assistance from NS proteins, including NS2 and NS5A. The HCV core protein forms the viral capsid through interactions with lipid droplets, p7, and the RNA genome. HCV glycoproteins E1 and E2 are transported to the surface of the HCV particle through the formation of a complex with NS2 and p7. After assembly within the ER, the HCV particle is released from the hepatocyte via the secretory pathway. The crystal structure of several potential targets for DAA therapy is depicted in **Fig. 4**.

As the HCV virus never enters the nucleus or integrates into the host genome, it is theoretically possible to eliminate HCV from the cytoplasm of the infected hepatocyte by blocking viral replication. Each step of the HCV life cycle serves as a potential target of direct-acting antivirals (DAAs). Through inhibition of specific viral proteins and other cellular components necessary for replication, therapy with DAAs has been able to more efficiently achieve replication arrest when compared with prior HCV therapies such an interferon. Moreover, as these viral proteins are unique to HCV, these targeted agents have improved safety and efficacy profiles when compared with prior interferon-based treatment regimens. Agents currently in development and those that have recently become approved have been shown to eliminate HCV RNA from the serum within hours to days of initial administration.

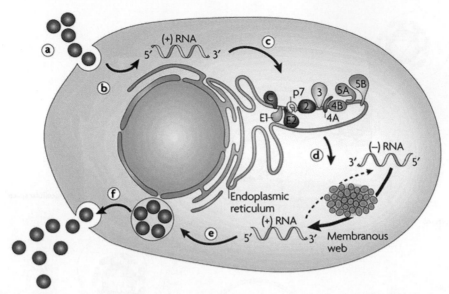

Fig. 2. Lifecycle of the HCV virus. Virus binding and internalization (a); cytoplasmic release and uncoating (b); IRES-mediated translation and polyprotein processing (c); RNA replication (d); packaging and assembly (e); virion maturation and release (f). IRES, internal ribosome entry site. (*From* Moradpour D, Penin F, Rice C. Replication of hepatitis C virus. Nat Rev Microbiol 2007;5:455; with permission.)

THE ISSUE OF POLYMORPHISMS AND DRUG RESISTANCE

Because of poor proofreading by the HCV RNA polymerase and rapid turnover of circulating virions, a complex mixture of different HCV variants or quasispecies exists.[12] HCV therapy may influence the emergence of resistant strains of virus as wild type virus is cleared; these resistant variants arise from pre-existing subpopulations

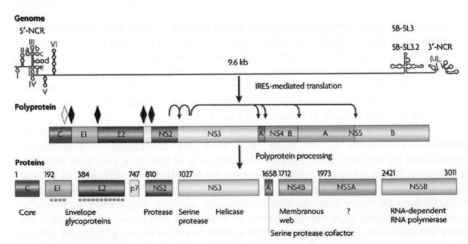

Fig. 3. The components of the HCV Genome after polyprotein processing. C, core; E, envelope; IRES, internal ribosome entry site; NCR, noncoding region; NS, nonstructural; SL, stemloop. (*From* Moradpour D, Penin F, Rice C. Replication of hepatitis C virus. Nat Rev Microbiol 2007;5:457; with permission.)

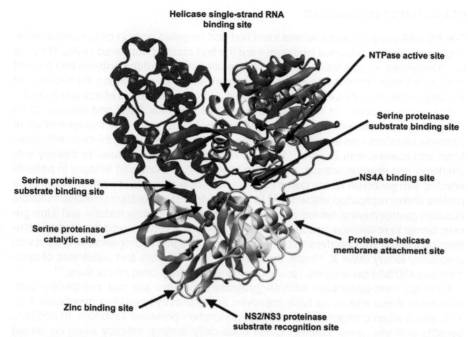

Fig. 4. The HCV and potential targets for DAAs. (*From* Pawlotsky JM, Chevaliez S, McHutchison JG. The hepatitis C virus life cycle as a target for new antiviral therapies. Gastroenterology 2007;132:1986; with permission.)

of virus that existed before therapy was initiated. The genetic barrier is the threshold at which the virus will mutate and replicate under selective pressure from a drug. A viral population with a low genetic barrier to resistance may have a pre-existing mutation, which does not impact viral fitness but rapidly emerges during therapy. A viral population with a high genetic barrier may require either a primary mutation that severely impacts viral fitness or several mutations in order to develop drug resistance. In addition, cross-resistance, in which a resistant mutation results in decreased sensitivity to a specific drug or class of DAA, may occur and influence future treatment options.[13]

An additional concern is the persistence of resistant mutations or resistance associated variants (RAVs). Theoretically, when HCV therapy is discontinued in patients who do not clear virus, the dominant population of virus that re-emerges is the more fit or wild-type virus, as the resistant HCV variants replicate less efficiently. However, the long-term survival or archiving of these resistant variants remains incompletely characterized. As DNA is not generated during HCV replication (in contradistinction to chronic human immunodeficiency virus [HIV] or hepatitis B virus [HBV] infection), the virus never enters the nucleus, and the resistant variants usually disappear over time; resistant mutations of HCV should not persist. As more accurate next-generation sequencing or ultradeep pyrosequencing assays to identify HCV resistance are developed, it is theoretically possible that persistent, low-level populations of resistant virus or RAVs may be identified in patients who fail to clear virus, affecting future treatment choices.[14] As a result, it is apparent that combination therapy with DAAs exhibiting a high barrier to resistance that target different segments of the HCV life cycle will be associated with a low risk of emergence of resistance and improved efficacy related to curing HCV infection.

NS3/4A PROTEASE INHIBITORS

The NS3/4A protease enzyme was identified and targeted early in drug development, and subsequently, protease inhibitors were the first class of approved DAAs. They are peptidomimetic agents that bind to the active catalytic site of the enzyme and prevent post-translational processing of the HCV polyprotein.[15] By preventing the cleavage of the polyprotein into its functional components, viral replication is effectively halted.

The crystal structure of the HCV proteases has been identified and appears to be morphologically different when comparing different genotypes. The first generation of protease inhibitors was specific to genotype 1 and was used in combination with interferon and ribavirin with improved virologic response when compared to therapy with interferon and ribavirin without a protease inhibitor.[16,17] Increased efficacy in patients infected with genotype 1b compared to 1a was noted, likely related to differing resistance profiles and/or replication efficiency.[18] Limitations to first-generation protease inhibitors included gastrointestinal issues, skin reactions, and bone marrow toxicity, and a low genetic barrier to resistance. In addition, first-generation protease inhibitors required combination therapy with interferon as well as ribavirin, a highly teratogenic compound with pregnancy safety class X. Finally, these agents are inhibitors and substrates of cytochrome p450 3A4 iso-enzyme, resulting in significant drug–drug interactions.[19]

Although next-generation NS3/4A protease inhibitors are not completely pan-genotypic, these agents do have improved antiviral activity against genotypes 1, 2, 4, 5, and 6 when compared with the first-generation protease inhibitors. In addition, benefits of these newer agents include once-daily dosing, efficacy when combined with other DAAs, and an improved safety profile including the fact that they are categorized as pregnancy classes B and C.[20] Second-generation NS3/4A protease inhibitors are being developed with pan-genotypic activity, including difficult-to-treat genotype 3, with a higher barrier to resistance when compared with first-generation protease inhibitors.[21]

The development of viral resistance or RAVs remains an issue with this class of DAAs, particularly the first generation of these agents, as resistant variants appear early in patients who experience virologic breakthrough. Newer protease inhibitors have a higher barrier to resistance compared with the first generation of these agents. All protease inhibitors bind to the active site of the NS3/4A protease, but as these compounds vary in structure (linear vs macrocyclic) and binding (covalent vs non-covalent), protease inhibitors have overlapping but distinct resistance profiles.[22] Naturally occurring populations or quasispecies of resistance mutations are uncommon, with the exception of the Q80K variant that is encountered in approximately 30% of patients with genotype 1a. This variant may affect response rates to simeprevir, particularly when this agent is utilized in combination with interferon and ribavirin. It has also been observed that under antiviral pressure, several protease resistance mutations have emerged in vivo. In particular, the R155K and A156T mutations have been shown to confer cross-resistance.[13] The presence of cross-resistance and long-term persistence of the mutations that emerged during therapy with earlier-generation agents may theoretically limit the ability to use newer generations of protease inhibitors against resistant variants.[19] However, there are limited data on the duration of these resistant strains and their impact on the efficacy of retreatment of protease inhibitor experienced patients who failed previous therapy.[22]

NS5A INHIBITORS

Although the exact role of NS5A in the HCV replication cycle remains incompletely understood, NS5A inhibitors have successfully demonstrated inhibition of viral synthesis and assembly.[10] Administration of NS5A inhibitors results in a biphasic decline in serum HCV RNA suggesting 2 modes of action.[23] NS5A inhibitors shift the distribution of NS5A proteins from the ER to lipid droplets, impeding the assembly and release of viral particles. The rapid decline of HCV RNA within the first 6 hours of administration is consistent with this mechanism of action. A slower, prolonged decline in HCV RNA follows as these drugs inhibit the formation of the membranous web necessary to create the replication complex. An additional putative mechanism of action is through prevention of hyperphosphorylation required for viral synthesis.[24]

NS5A inhibitors are pan-genotypic; however, first-generation NS5A inhibitors do not display similar antiviral activity against all genotypes.[25] Additional benefits of these agents include a long half-life and high potency, making once-daily dosing possible. Overall, these drugs have been well tolerated with rare reported serious adverse events.[26,27] Several NS5A inhibitors are substrates of CYP3A4 and have a moderate risk of drug–drug interactions. Currently available NS5A inhibitors have a pregnancy class B, although other NS5A inhibitors in development have shown reproductive toxicity in animal studies.

There are pre-existing resistance mutations or RAV's to NS5A inhibitors that may emerge with successful suppression of wild-type virus. Monotherapy with NS5A inhibitors results in viral breakthrough in vivo with the same resistant mutations found in vitro. The most common substitutions occurred at positions M28, Q30, L31, H58, and Y93 in the NS5A sequence, and combination mutations such as Q30R-H58D conferred the highest level of resistance. These mutations occur more commonly in genotype 1a compared with genotype 1b.[28] Resistant strains appear to persist after therapy is discontinued, implying a higher degree of viral fitness.[29] Despite the low barrier to resistance with the first-generation NS5A inhibitors, no cross-resistance to other classes of DAA has been discovered; therefore, several successful DAA combinations include NS5As as part of the regimen.

NS5B POLYMERASE INHIBITORS

NS5B polymerase is the key enzyme responsible for HCV synthesis and is successfully targeted by 2 separate mechanisms. NS5B polymerase inhibitors exist as both nucleoside/nucleotide analogues and nonnucleoside inhibitors. The polymerase has a highly conserved active catalytic site that is stable across all genotypes, as well as 4 allosteric inhibitor-binding sites, domains known as thumb I/II, palm I/II. The active site is inhibited by nucleoside/nucleotide inhibitors, while non-nucleoside inhibitors act on the allosteric-binding sites, resulting in conformational change of the enzyme. Drugs targeting the HCV polymerase are highly selective with generally minimal toxicity due to the absence of a human counterpart.

Nucleoside/Nucleotide Analogue Inhibitors of Hepatitis C Virus NS5B Polymerase

A nucleoside is a base bound to a sugar, while a nucleotide is a base bound to a phosphate group. Nucleoside and nucleotide inhibitors are analogues of the natural substrates required for viral replication, and are incorporated into newly synthesized HCV RNA, resulting in chain termination and replication arrest. Nucleoside/nucleotide inhibitors are prodrugs that require triphosphorylation within the hepatocyte to become active.[30] In studies of viral kinetics, administration of nucleoside inhibitors resulted in a slow initial decline in HCV RNA. This phenomenon may be related to initial phosphorylation serving as a rate-limiting step, or a delay in accumulation of intracellular nucleoside triphosphates.[31] Antiviral effectiveness improves with twice-daily dosing. In comparison, nucleotide analogues only require 2 phosphorylation steps within the hepatocyte to become active at the target site, resulting in a more rapid decline in HCV.[32] Drug–drug interactions may occur with nucleoside/nucleotide analogues when combined with drugs that inhibit or induce the p-glycoprotein transporter or other nucleoside analogues such as chemotherapeutic or antiviral agents.[33] Based on animal data, the currently approved nucleotide inhibitor sofosbuvir has a pregnancy safety class B rating.

NS5B is a key enzyme of HCV RNA synthesis, and its active site is highly-conserved. As a result, drugs targeting this site have pan-genotypic activity and a high barrier to resistance.[34] The emergence of resistant strains in uncommon, as even if these variants emerge, they have poor viral fitness.[35] The most common mutation identified at the active site of NS5B is S282T, which may be a pre-existing mutation or emerge during treatment. However, this variant has diminished fitness and replicates at a much lower rate when compared with wild-type virus.[36] In a small subset of patients, certain NS5B substitutions (L159F, V321A, C316A, and S282R) have emerged during nucleoside/nucleotide inhibitor therapy, resulting in treatment failure that may potentially alter future treatment choices.[37] These mutant variants may result in cross-resistance to this class of drugs, but currently, their significance remains unknown.

NON-NUCLEOSIDE INHIBITORS OF HEPATITIS C VIRUS NS5B POLYMERASE

Non-nucleoside inhibitors (NNI) bind to one of four allosteric sites on the polymerase, resulting in conformational change in the enzyme and indirectly halting RNA synthesis. The HCV RdRp has a right-hand shape with allosteric binding sites located in the thumb and palm domains (**Fig. 5**).

Compared with the active catalytic site targeted by the nucleoside/nucleotide analogues, these regions are less conserved and are susceptible to variations across genotypes. As a result, NNIs are predominantly specific to genotype 1a/1b and have a low barrier to resistance. Some agents appear to be less effective against genotype 1a compared with genotype 1b.[38] The thumb I and II domains have a unique set of

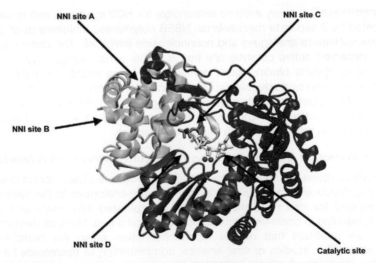

Fig. 5. Ribbon diagram of the HCV RNA-dependent RNA polymerase. The fingers, palm and thumb subdomains are colored in blue, red, and green, respectively. (*From* Pawlotsky JM, Chevaliez S, McHutchison JG. The hepatitis C virus life cycle as a target for new antiviral therapies. Gastroenterology 2007;132:1988; with permission.)

Table 1
HCV DAA's pros and cons

	Genotypes	Potency	Barrier to Resistance	Drug–Drug Interactions	Toxicity	Pharmacokinentics	Teratogenicity
NS3/4A Protease inhibitors							
First generation	Variable 1, 4, 6	High	Low 1a<1b (Q80K)	High	First generation: rash anemia, gastrointestinal	Daily to three times daily	Variable Class B, C
Second generation	1–6				Second generation: fatigue, photosensitivity, rash, gastrointestinal		
NS5A inhibitors							
First generation	Variable 1, 4	High	Low 1a<1b	Low–moderate	Low: fatigue, nausea, headache	Daily	Variable
Second generation	1, 4>2, 3						
Nucleoside/nucleotide inhibitors	1–6	Moderate/high	Very high	Low	Fatigue, headache	Daily to twice daily	Class B
Non-nucleoside inhibitors	Variable	Variable	Very low 1a<1b	Moderate	Fatigue Nausea Pruritus	Daily to three times daily	Class B

resistant mutations, while the palm sites I and II have partially overlapping resistance profiles.[39] Palm II inhibitors are unique in this class in that they are active against genotypes 1 to 4. Mutations at NS5B M423 and S556 are associated with treatment failure.[40,41] Despite these limitations, NNIs are effective against resistance mutations that emerge after therapy with other classes of DAAs, and the absence of cross-resistance makes NNIs good candidates for combination therapy with other DAAs.

Similar to nucleoside/nucleotide analogues, NNIs are substrates of the P-glycoprotein transporter, and drug interactions may occur. Additionally, the currently available NNI dasabuvir is metabolized by CYP2C8, and increased levels may occur when paired with an inhibitor of this enzyme.[42] Toxicity related to NNIs consists mostly of gastrointestinal and dermatologic events.[5] Based on current data from animal studies, no increased risk in pregnancy has been found (pregnancy class B).

THE RATIONALE BEHIND COMBINATION THERAPY

In order for a DAA to be an ideal candidate as a component of HCV therapy, it should demonstrate a high barrier to resistance, pan-genotypic activity, and high potency. Currently, nucleotide analogue inhibitors are considered the backbone of DAA therapy, as they meet all of these criteria, and have shown to successfully achieve viral eradication when combined with several different classes of DAAs, including protease inhibitors, NS5A inhibitors, or NNIs.[36] High potency, elevated barrier to resistance, and pan-genotypic activity also allow nucleotide analogues to be combined with 1 additional agent to achieve successful eradication of HCV. In addition, the relative paucity of drug–drug interactions and ability to coformulate these agents with an additional DAA improve both tolerability and adherence to therapy. As second-generation potent and pan-genotypic protease inhibitors with a high barrier to resistance become available, they may soon also serve as a backbone for combination therapy.

Antiviral combinations that do not include a nucleotide analogue inhibitor must combat the risk of viral breakthrough due to emergence of resistant mutations.[43] Therefore, regimens containing less potent drugs with a lower barrier to resistance generally require 3 or more drugs to be combined in order to prevent viral breakthrough and relapse due to the emergence of multidrug resistant subtypes.[15] As an example, a recently approved regimen containing a ritonavir-boosted protease inhibitor, nonnucleoside polymerase inhibitor, and an NS5A inhibitor has been developed. Ribavirin needs to be added to this regimen to optimize response rates in genotype 1a patients.[41] This regimen is effective with low-level post-therapy viral relapse and on therapy viral breakthrough, but illustrates the requirement for DAAs of several different classes if the regimen does not contain a nucleoside inhibitor.

An additional consideration relating to combining DAAs relates to the ability to shorten therapy when combining different agents. Recently published data have demonstrated near-universal viral cure in HCV genotype 1-infected patients when combining a potent nucleoside polymerase inhibitor, NS5A inhibitor, and either a protease inhibitor or non-nucleoside polymerase inhibitor with only 6 weeks of therapy.[44] It is clear that the optimal combinations of DAA will continue to evolve as new, more potent agents become approved.

SUMMARY

The approval of all-oral DAA therapy has been associated with a revolution in the management of HCV, with the ability to achieve nearly universal eradication of viral replication in the vast majority of patients. These agents have various strengths and weaknesses, outlined in **Table 1**. The availability of multiple different classes of agents presents an opportunity to optimize therapy by combining potent, pan-genotypic agents with a high barrier to resistance to achieve rapid and safe eradication of virus. The optimal treatment algorithm continues to evolve as new agents enter the treatment armamentarium; however, it is conceivable that the ability to achieve HCV eradication in all varieties of HCV-infected patients will become a reality.

REFERENCES

1. Merz A, Long G, Hiet M, et al. Biochemical and morphological properties of hepatitis C virus particles and determination of their lipidome. J Biol Chem 2011;286: 3018–32.
2. Chang K, Jiang J, Cai Z, et al. Human apolipoprotein E is required for infectivity and production of hepatitis C virus in cell culture. J Virol 2007;81:13783–93.
3. Dubuisson J, Cosset FL. Virology and cell biology of the hepatitis C virus life cycle- an update. J Hepatol 2014;61:S3–7.
4. Pileri P, Uematsu Y, Campagnoli G, et al. Binding of hepatitis C virus to CD81. Science 1998;282:938–41.
5. Zeisel M, Felmlee D, Baumert T. Hepatitis C virus entry. Curr Top Microbiol Immunol 2013;369:87–112.
6. Ashfaq U, Javed T, Rehman S, et al. An overview of HCV molecular biology, replication and immune responses. J Virol 2011;8:161–71.
7. Albecka A, Belouzard S, Op de Beeck A, et al. Role of low-density lipoprotein receptor in the hepatitis C virus life cycle. Hepatology 2012;55:998–1007.
8. Moradpour D, Penin F, Rice C. Replication of hepatitis C virus. Nat Rev Microbiol 2007;5:453–63.
9. Pawlotsky JM, Chevaliez S, McHutchison JG. The hepatitis C virus life cycle as a target for new antiviral therapies. Gastroenterology 2007;132:1979–98.
10. Kohler JJ, Nettles JH, Amblard F, et al. Approaches to hepatitis C treatment and cure using NS5A inhibitors. Infect Drug Resist 2014;7:41–56.
11. Gerold G, Pietschmann T. The HCV life cycle: in vitro tissue culture systems and therapeutic targets. Dig Dis 2014;32:525–37.
12. Halfon P, Locarnini S. Hepatitis C viral resistance to protease inhibitors. J Hepatol 2011;55:192–206.
13. Halfon P, Sarrazin C. Future treatment of chronic hepatitis C with direct acting antivirals: is resistance important? Liver Int 2012;32:79–87.
14. Ji H, Kozak RA, Biondi MJ, et al. Next generation sequencing of the hepatitis C virus NS5B gene reveals potential novel S282 drug resistance mutations. Virology 2015;16(477C):1–9.
15. Pawlotsky JM. New hepatitis C therapies: the toolbox, strategies, and challenges. Gastroenterology 2014;466:1176–92.
16. McHutchison J, Everson G, Gordon S, et al. Telaprevir with peginterferon and ribavirin for chronic HCV genotype 1 infection. N Engl J Med 2009;360:1827–38.
17. Poordad F, McCone JJ, Bacon B, et al. Boceprevir for untreated chronic HCV genotype 1 infection. N Engl J Med 2011;364:1195–206.
18. Wyles D, Gutierrez J. Importance of HCV genotype 1 subtypes for drug resistance and response to therapy. J Viral Hepat 2014;21:229–40.
19. De Luca A, Bianco C, Rossetti B. Treatment of HCV infection with the novel NS3/4A protease inhibitors. Curr Opin Pharmacol 2014;8:9–17.
20. Clark V, Peter JA, Nelson DR. New therapeutic strategies in HCV: second generation protease inhibitors. Liver Int 2013;33:80–4.

21. Harper S, Jan M, Rudd M, et al. Discovery of MK-5172, a macrocyclic hepatitis C virus NS3/4a protease inhibitor. ACS Med Chem Lett 2012;3:332–6.
22. Kieffer TL, George S. Resistance to hepatitis C virus protease inhibitors. Curr Opin Virol 2014;8:16–21.
23. Guedj J, Dahari H, Rong L, et al. Modeling shows that the NS5A inhibitor daclatasvir has two modes of action and yields a shorter estimate of the hepatitis C virus half-life. Proc Natl Acad Sci U S A 2013;110:3991–6.
24. Pawlotsky J. NS5A inhibitors in the treatment of hepatitis C. J Hepatol 2013;59:375–82.
25. Gao M. Antiviral activity and resistance of HCV NS5A replication complex inhibitors. Curr Opin Virol 2013;3:514–20.
26. Afdhal N, Zeuzem S, Kwo P, et al. Ledipasvir and sofosbuvir for untreated HCV genotype 1 infection. N Engl J Med 2014;370:1889–98.
27. Sulkowski MS, Jacobson IM, Nelson DR. Daclatasvir plus sofosbuvir for previously treated or untreated chronic HCV infection. N Engl J Med 2014;370:211–21.
28. Fridell R, Wang C, Sun J, et al. Genotypic and phenotypic analysis of variants resistant to hepatitis C virus nonstructural protein 5A replication complex inhibitor BMS-790052 in humans: invitro and invivo correlations. Hepatology 2011;54:1924–35.
29. McPhee F, Hernandez D, Yu F, et al. Resistance analysis of hepatitis C virus genotype 1 prior treatment null responders receiving daclatasvir and asunaprevir. Hepatology 2013;58:902–11.
30. Bhatia H, Singh H, Grewal N, et al. Sofosbuvir: a novel treatment option for chronic hepatitis C infection. J Pharmacol Pharmacother 2014;5:278–84.
31. Guedj J, Dahari H, Shudo E, et al. Hepatitis C viral kinetics with the nucleoside polymerase inhibitor mericitabine (RG7128). Hepatology 2012;55:1030–7.
32. Guedj J, Pang PD, Rodriguez-Torres M, et al. Analysis of hepatitis C viral kinetics during administration of two nucleotide analogues: sofosbuvir (GS-7977) and GS-0938. Antivir Ther 2014;19:211–20.
33. Soriano V, Labarga P, Barreiro PF. Drug interactions with new hepatitis C oral drugs. Expert Opin Drug Metab Toxicol 2015;2:1–9.
34. Schmidt W, Nelson D, Pawlotsky J, et al. Direct-acting antiviral agents and the path to interferon independence. Clin Gastroenterol Hepatol 2014;12:728–37.
35. Svarovskaia E, Dvory-Sobol H, Parkin N, et al. Infrequent development of resistance in genotype 1–6 hepatitis C virus-infected subjected treated with sofosbuvir in phase 2 and 3 clinical trials. Clin Infect Dis 2014;59:1666–74.
36. Bourliere M, Oules V, Ansaldi C, et al. Sofosbuvir as backbone of interferon free treatments. Dig Liver Dis 2014;15:S212–220.
37. Donaldson E, Harrington P, O'Rear J, et al. Clinicalaepatitis C virus resistance pathways for sofosbuvir. Hepatology 2015;61:56–65.
38. Zeuzem S, Soriano V, Asselah T, et al. Faldaprevir and deleobuvir for HCV genotype 1 infection. N Engl J Med 2013;369:630–9.
39. Kati W, Koev G, Irvin M, et al. In vitro activity and resistance profile of dasabuvir, a non-nucleoside HCV polymerase inhibitor. Antimicrob Agents Chemother 2014;22:1–27.
40. Fenaux M, Eng S, Leavitt SA, et al. Preclinical characterization of GS-9669, a thumb site II inhibitor of the hepatitis C virus NS5B polymerase. Antimicrob Agents Chemother 2013;57:804–10.
41. Feld J, Kowdley K, Coakley E, et al. Treatment of HCV with ABT-450/r-ombitasvir and dasabuvir with ribavirin. N Engl J Med 2014;370:1594–603.

42. Gentile I, Buonomo A, Borgia G. Dasabuvir: a non-nucleoside inhibitor of NS5B for the treatment of hepatitis C virus infection. Rev Recent Clin Trials 2014;9(2): 115–23.
43. Welzel T, Dultz G, Zeuzem S. Interferon-free antiviral combination therapies without nucleosidic polymerase inhibitors. J Hepatol 2014;61:S98–107.
44. Kohli A, Osinusi A, Sims Z, et al. Virological response after 6 week triple-drug regimens for hepatitis C: a proof-of-concept phase 2A cohort study. Lancet 2015; 385(9973):1107–13.

Regimens for the Hepatitis C Treatment-Naive Patient

Walid S. Ayoub, MD[a,b,*], Tram T. Tran, MD[b]

KEYWORDS

- Interferon-free • Treatment naive • Cirrhosis • DAA • Direct acting antivirals

KEY POINTS

- Multiple ongoing clinical trials with various direct-acting antivirals (DAAs) are demonstrating high efficacy combined with shorter duration of treatment and good tolerability.
- The success of these advancements allowed the elimination of interferon-based therapy for hepatitis C virus (HCV) infection.
- Future treatments of hepatitis C will consist of all oral regimens that combine agents of different classes that will result in pangenotypic coverage and shorter duration of treatment.
- There are numerous clinical trials, with next-generation DAAs already showing promise in shortening therapy, with no impact on sustained virologic response (SVR).

INTRODUCTION

HCV infection is a leading cause of cirrhosis and hepatocellular carcinoma globally. Most individuals infected with HCV are asymptomatic and often unaware of their infection. It is estimated that 160 million persons are infected with hepatitis C worldwide.[1] Recent recommendations in the United States targeting screening of Baby Boomers, adults born between 1945 and 1965, is expected to have a positive impact on reducing the burden of hepatitis C by identifying more infected individuals for therapy. Although treatment success during the era of interferon-based therapy was between 40% and 80%, the introduction of the newer DAA therapies has led to achievement of treatment success rates of more than 90%. A sustained virological response (SVR) is

Disclosures: Dr W. Ayoub, MD, served on advisory boards for BMS, Abbvie and Gilead. He receives research grants from BMS and Gilead. Dr. T. Tran, MD, is a speaker/consultant for Gilead, Abbvie, BMS and Jansen. She receives research grants from Gilead and BMS and is an advisor for Gilead, BMS, Abbvie and Jansen.
[a] Department of Gastroenterology, Cedars Sinai Medical Center, 8730 Alden Drive, Suite E235, Los Angeles, CA 90048, USA; [b] Liver Transplant Program, Cedars Sinai Medical Center, 8900 Beverly Boulevard, Suite 250, Los Angeles, CA 90048, USA
* Corresponding author. Liver Transplant Program, 8900 Beverly Boulevard, Suite 250, Los Angeles, CA 90048.
E-mail address: Walid.Ayoub@cshs.org

the end point of therapy. Once achieved, SVR is considered a virologic cure and is defined as undetectable HCV RNA 12 weeks after end of therapy (SVR12). Achieving SVR12 is associated with resolution of liver disease in patients without cirrhosis and reduction in the rates of complications from cirrhosis and portal hypertension in patients with cirrhosis.[2] This article reviews current approved non–interferon-based therapy and data from clinical trials in treatment-naive patients with chronic HCV infection.

Currently available DAA therapy is divided into 3 main classes: protease (NS3/4) inhibitors, NS5A inhibitors, and polymerase inhibitors (NS5B) nucleosides/nucleotides (nucs) and nonnucleotide polymerase inhibitors. The protease inhibitors are characterized by their high potency, limited genotypic coverage, and low barrier to resistance. The NS5A inhibitors have high potency, multigenotypic coverage, and low barrier to resistance. The NS5B nucleotide inhibitors have intermediate potency, pangenotypic coverage, and high barrier to resistance, whereas the NS5B nonnucleotide polymerase inhibitors have intermediate potency, limited genotypic coverage, and low barrier to resistance (**Tables 1** and **2**). Unlike interferon-based therapy, DAA therapy has overcome many of the poor prognostic indicators for reduced SVR rates; however, with newer therapies comes the need for understanding new issues of viral resistance factors, potential side effects, and drug-drug interactions and virologic factors that were predictive of lower SVR rates.[3]

TREATMENT IN NAIVE PATIENTS WITHOUT CIRRHOSIS
Hepatitis C Virus Genotype 1

Multiple approved regimens are available for the treatment of treatment-naive patients with HCV genotype 1 infection. Sofosbuvir-based combination therapy has been studied extensively as one of the foundations of new DAA-based therapy. The ELECTRON study was a phase 2 clinical trial that provided early proof of concept that interferon-free therapy was possible for the treatment of chronic hepatitis C. One arm of the ELECTRON study had 25 treatment-naive patients who achieved an SVR rate of 84% with a combination of sofosbuvir and ribavirin for 12 weeks regardless of the IL28B T-allele.[4] Compared with the ELECTRON trial, the phase 2 SPARE trial was a randomized, open-label, 2-part, phase 2 study that proved that SVR can be improved with prolonged therapy even in patients with typically unfavorable treatment characteristics (men, African Americans, IL28B-non CC, HCV genotype 1a (HCV-1a) infection, and cirrhosis in 23% of the population). Patients were given sofosbuvir and weight-based ribavirin (1000 mg [<75 kg] to 1200 mg [≥75 kg]) for 24 weeks in part 1 of the SPARE trial, and SVR was reported as 90% (9 of 10). However, in part 2 of this study, in which weight-based dose of ribavirin in combination with sofosbuvir was given, the SVR rate was subsequently only 68% (17 of 25) compared with 48% (12 of 25) in patients receiving low fixed-dose ribavirin in conjunction with sofosbuvir.[5] The QUANTUM study, another phase 2b trial, showed an SVR of 47% and 53% in treatment-naive patients treated for 12 or 24 weeks, respectively.[6]

Table 1			
Characteristics of the direct-acting antiviral agents			
	Potency	Genotypic Coverage	Barrier to Resistance
NS3/4 protease inhibitors	High	Limited	Low
NS5A inhibitors	High	Multigenotypic	Low
NS5B nucs	Intermediate	Pangenotypic	High
NS5B Non-nucs	Intermediate	Limited	Low

Table 2			
Classes of the direct-acting antiviral therapy			
N3/4 Protease Inhibitors	NS5A Inhibitors	Nuc Polymerase Inhibitors	Non-Nuc Polymerase Inhibitors
Paritaprevir	Ombitasvir	—	Dasabuvir
Grazoprevir	Elbasvir	—	—
Simeprevir	Daclatasvir	—	—
—	GS-5816	Sofosbuvir	—
—	Ledipasvir	—	—

Sofosbuvir/ledipasvir (SOF/LDV), a combination of the NS5B nucleotide inhibitor sofosbuvir and the NS5A inhibitor ledipasvir, was approved in the United States in 2015 based on the ION-1 and ION-3 registration trials. ION-1 contained 726 treatment-naive patients and ION-3 had 647 patients. Of the patients in the ION-1 trial, 67% had HCV-1a infection. The addition of ribavirin or extending the duration from 12 to 24 weeks with SOF/LDV did not affect SVR12. The SVR12 was 97% to 99%. Race was not found to be a factor for response as 98% of whites, 100% blacks, and 100% Hispanics achieved SVR in the ION-1 trial.[7] ION-3 was a large open-label randomized study designed to compare 8 weeks (SOF/LDV/ribavirin or SOF/LDV) with 12 weeks of treatment (SOF/LDV). The SVR12 rates were 93% to 94% and 95% in the 8- and 12-week arms, respectively, with and without ribavirin. However, the relapse rate was higher in the 8-week arm (20 of 431) than in the 12-week arm (3 of 216) regardless of the addition of ribavirin. Post hoc analysis revealed that a low HCV viral load defined as less than 6 million IU/mL was associated with a similar relapse rate of 2% in the 8- and 12-week arms.[8] However, because the post hoc analysis was not controlled, the American Association for the Study of Liver Diseases (AASLD) and Infectious Diseases Society of America (IDSA) guidelines recommend caution with shortening the duration of therapy to less than 12 weeks.[3]

Paritaprevir/ritonavir/ombitasvir plus dasabuvir (also referred to as the 3D regimen) and weight-based ribavirin is the latest approved DAA therapy for the treatment of HCV genotype 1 infection. Unlike SOF/LDV, the use of ribavirin with the 3D regimen depends on the HCV subgenotype and the level of fibrosis. SAPPHIRE-1 was an international phase 3, placebo-controlled clinical trial, which included 322 treatment-naive noncirrhotic patients with HCV-1a infection who were treated with 12 weeks of 3D regimen with weight-based ribavirin. SVR12 was 95.3% in HCV-1a infection and 98% in HCV genotype 1b (HCV-1b) infection. Stepwise logistic regression found no impact of age, sex, fibrosis score, and baseline viral load on the SVR12. Only the body mass index (BMI) was associated with slightly reduced rate with an odds ratio of 0.89 ($P = .02$). However, SVR12 was still 91.5% among patients with BMI 30 or more.[9] PEARL-IV was another phase 3 clinical trial that included 419 patients with HCV-1b infection and 305 patients with HCV-1a infection that randomized patients to receive 3D regimen with and without ribavirin. SVR12 was unaffected by the use of ribavirin in the HCV-1b group (99.5% with ribavirin vs 99% without ribavirin). The addition of ribavirin had a greater impact on SVR12 in patients with HCV-1a infection. Adding ribavirin yielded an SVR of 97% compared with an SVR of 90.2% in the group without ribavirin. Therefore, the virologic failure rate was higher in the HCV-1a group without ribavirin (7.8%) compared with the group that received ribavirin (2%) because of relapse.[10] As a result, the US Food and Drug Administration (FDA) label for this combination requires the use of ribavirin in patients with HCV-1a infection.

The combination of sofosbuvir and simeprevir (SOF/SIM) was first studied in 40 naive patients with HCV infection with advanced fibrosis (F3-F4) in the COSMOS trial.[11] Two recently reported real-world databases (HCV-TARGET and TRIO) addressed the use and outcome of such therapy. The HCV-TARGET is a multicenter international registry that involves both academic and community centers. It included 323 patients with HCV genotype 1 infection who were treatment naive and without cirrhosis. The results of the SVR, 4 weeks after end of treatment (SVR4), of the HCV-TARGET were presented at the AASLD meeting in 2014. The SVR4 was 87% in all naive patients with HCV genotype 1 infection treated with SOF/SIM and 89% in the SOF/SIM/ribavirin group.[12] Overall, patients with genotype 1b infection did better (SVR4, 92%–93%) than patients with genotype 1a infection (SVR4, 82%–84%). There were no presented data on the results of the treatment-naive patients based on presence or absence of cirrhosis. The TRIO study also reported its prospective observational cohort of treated patients with HCV infection from US academic medical centers and community physicians in partnership with a specialty pharmacy. An SVR12 of 99% was achieved in treatment-naive and noncirrhotic patients.[13]

The combination of sofosbuvir and daclatasvir, another NS5A inhibitor, for 12 weeks is currently approved in Europe for the treatment of naive patients with chronic HCV genotype 1 infection. However, such therapy is not yet approved in the United States. Preliminary data reported that both 12-week (n = 14) and 24-week (n = 41) treatment course of therapy resulted in an SVR12 of 100%.[14] Phase 3 registration studies of this regimen are underway.

Hepatitis C Virus Genotype 2

The currently approved treatment of patients with HCV genotype 2 infection is a combination of sofosbuvir and weight-based dose of ribavirin for 12 weeks in treatment-naive patients without cirrhosis. The FISSION trial addressed the use of 12 weeks of sofosbuvir and ribavirin therapy in 73 patients with HCV genotype 2 infection. The SVR rate was 95%. When taking cirrhosis into account, the SVR rate was better in noncirrhotic patients (97%) than in cirrhotic patients (83%).[15] The POSITRON trial included interferon ineligible patients who were also treated with 12 weeks of sofosbuvir and ribavirin with an SVR of 93%.[16] More support for the treatment of patients with HCV genotype 2 infection came with the release of the VALENCE study. The VALENCE study is a phase 3, multicenter, international clinical trial. It included treatment-naive and experienced patients. Among patients with HCV genotype 2 infection (G2) who received 12 weeks of sofosbuvir-ribavirin, 68 of 73 (93%; 95% confidence interval [CI], 85–98) had an SVR 12 weeks after the cessation of treatment, with 93.7% SVR in the noncirrhotic patients with G2 and 81.8% in the cirrhotic patients with G2 studied.[17] Subanalysis of the treatment-naive group without cirrhosis revealed an SVR12 of 96.7% (29 of 30).[17] Real-life data from the TRIO health study as presented at the AASLD reported an SVR12 of 90%. However, presented data did not separate cirrhotic from noncirrhotic patients.[13] It is notable that no virologic breakthroughs were observed in treatment-adherent patients and there was no relationship between relapse and the selection of resistant HCV variants in the reported studies.

Hepatitis C Virus Genotype 3

The only currently approved regimen in the United States for the treatment of HCV genotype 3 infection is a 24-week regimen of sofosbuvir and weight-based dose of ribavirin. This regimen is associated with an SVR of 91% in treatment-naive patients.[17]

Shorter regimen of 12 weeks was studied in the FISSION trial. However, such approach yielded a disappointing overall SVR of 56% (102 of 183). As expected, the response rate was better in noncirrhotic patients (61%).[15] Extending therapy to 16 weeks did not yield much better results according to the FUSION trial, as SVR was only achieved in only 62% of cases.[16] The VALENCE trial yielded a better result with prolongation of therapy to 24 weeks as 94% (86 of 92) of patients achieved SVR12 with 24 weeks of sofosbuvir and ribavirin therapy.[17] No virologic breakthroughs were observed in treatment-adherent patients. In addition, there was no relationship between relapse and the selection of resistant HCV variants.

TREATMENT IN NAIVE PATIENTS WITH CIRRHOSIS
Hepatitis C Virus Genotype 1

The combination of sofosbuvir and simeprevir was one of the first combination therapies used for the treatment of HCV infection without interferon in the COSMOS trial. COSMOS was a phase 2 trial that included cirrhotic and noncirrhotic patients. Cohort 2 of the study included treatment-naive and null-responder patients with F3-F4 fibrosis. The combination of sofosbuvir and simeprevir for 12 weeks yielded an SVR of 86% (6 of 7) in naive patients with F4 fibrosis compared with 100% SVR in patients (10 of 10) treated for 24 weeks.[11] It was not surprising that the FDA subsequently recommended 24 weeks of treatment in all patients with cirrhosis. Real life data on the use of such combination therapy came from the HCV-TARGET and TRIO health studies. The HCV-TARGET revealed an overall SVR4 in patients with cirrhosis of 85% regardless of prior treatment status. Subanalysis of the findings revealed an SVR4 of 82% in patients with HCV-1a infection compared with SVR4 of 87% in patients with HCV-1b infection.[12] The TRIO Health study also shed light on the efficacy of treatment based on sofosbuvir and simeprevir in cirrhotic patients in the community and at academic centers. It revealed an overall SVR12 of 85% with the use of the combination of sofosbuvir and simeprevir with or without ribavirin.[13] However, no specific data were presented on the treatment-naive patients.

The fixed-dose combination of SOF/LDV is also efficacious in the treatment of patients with HCV-1a and HCV-1b infection. The approved therapy is for 12 weeks in naive patients with cirrhosis.[3] The ION-1 phase 3 clinical trial included 136 cirrhotic patients. The trial also demonstrated equal efficacy of the therapy in HCV subgenotypes 1a versus 1b infection and in white, black, and Hispanic patients. The rate of SVR12 in patients with cirrhosis was 94% to 100% based on an intention-to-treat analysis of the trial.[7]

Ombitasvir/paritaprevir/ritonavir and dasabuvir (the 3D regimen) with ribavirin was also studied in the TURQUOISE II, a phase 3 randomized, open-label, international trial. The study randomized treatment-naive and cirrhotic patients with Child-Turcotte-Pugh class A cirrhosis to 12 or 24 weeks of treatment. The SVR12 in the naive cirrhotic patients was 94.2% and 94.6% with 12 and 24 weeks, respectively.[18]

Hepatitis C Virus Genotype 2

The recommended treatment of cirrhotic patients with HCV genotype 2 is 16[3,19] or 20[19] weeks of therapy with sofosbuvir and weight-based dose of ribavirin. The 20% cirrhotic patients of the FISSION trial treated with sofosbuvir and ribavirin for 12 weeks achieved an SVR of 72%.[15] The FUSION trial compared 12 and 16 weeks regimen in patients with cirrhosis. The SVR rate was better with the prolonged therapy to 16 weeks compared with 12 weeks at 78% (7 of 9) and 60% (6 of 10), respectively.[16] This finding is the basis for the consideration of longer duration of therapy than

12 weeks in patients with cirrhosis. The VALENCE trial included 11 cirrhotic patients with HCV-2 who were treated with sofosbuvir and ribavirin for 12 weeks leading to an SVR12 of 81.8% (9 of 11). However, it only included 2 treatment-naive patients of the 11 patients with cirrhosis. Both patients were treated with sofosbuvir and ribavirin and achieved an SVR12.[17] However, a lower rate of response was noted in the real-world data from the TRIO Health.[13] More data will be emerging regarding the optimal duration of treatment of patients with cirrhosis and HCV-2 because the registration trials included few patients with cirrhosis and HCV genotype 2.

Hepatitis C Virus Genotype 3

The recommended treatment of treatment-naive patients with hepatitis C genotype 3 infection and cirrhosis is 24 weeks of therapy with sofosbuvir and ribavirin. Cirrhotic patients of the FISSION trials who received sofosbuvir and ribavirin for 12 weeks had an SVR12 of only 34% (13 of 38).[15] Extending therapy to 24 weeks in the VALENCE trial with sofosbuvir and ribavirin yielded an SVR12 of 68.3% (41 of 60) in cirrhotic patients. When considering only the treatment-naive patients with cirrhosis, a better SVR of 92% (12 of 13) was noted.[17] Four factors were independently associated with an SVR in this trial: a baseline HCV RNA level of less than $6 \log_{10}$ IU/mL (odds ratio, 4.23; 95% CI, 1.21–14.81; $P = .02$), female sex (odds ratio, 3.18; 95% CI, 1.22–8.31; $P = .02$), absence of cirrhosis (odds ratio, 3.46; 95% CI, 1.60–7.48; $P = .002$), and an age of less than 50 years (odds ratio, 2.82; 95% CI, 1.21–6.57; $P = .02$).[17] More effective therapy is expected to emerge in the near future for this population.

TREATMENT OF HEPATITIS C VIRUS GENOTYPE 4 INFECTION

Three options are available for the treatment of patients with HCV genotype 4 infection according to the AASLD/IDSA: SOF/LDV for 12 weeks, 3D regimen with ribavirin for 12 weeks, and sofosbuvir with weight-based ribavirin for 24 weeks.

The Synergy trial is an open-label study that evaluated 12 weeks' therapy using SOF/LDV in 21 patients. About 60% of the patients were treatment naive, and 57% were noncirrhotic patients. Preliminary analysis revealed an SVR12 of 95% by intention-to-treat analysis and 100% by per-protocol analysis.[20]

PEARL-I, an open-label phase 2b study, also addressed therapy in 86 treatment-naive patients with HCV genotype 4 infection and with and without cirrhosis using paritaprevir/ritonavir/ombitasvir with or without ribavirin for 12 weeks. The addition of ribavirin yielded better SVR12 of 100% (42 of 42) compared with 90.9% (40 of 44) without the addition of ribavirin.[21]

The use of sofosbuvir with ribavirin in patients with HCV genotype 4 infection has been supported in multiple studies. A small US study addressed the use of 12 and 24 weeks of sofosbuvir and ribavirin in 80 patients of Egyptian descent. Fourteen patients were treatment naive in each arm of the study. As with HCV genotype 3 infection, prolonged duration of treatment resulted in an improved SVR12 of 79% (11 of 14) in the 12-week arm compared with SVR12 of 100% (14 of 14) in the 24-week arm. Patients with cirrhosis were significantly disadvantaged with 12 weeks of therapy, as SVR12 was achieved only in 43% (3 of 7) of the cases compared with an SVR12 of 100% (7 of 7) with 24 weeks of therapy.[22] A larger phase 2 clinical trial performed in Egypt also found similar results. A 24-week course of sofosbuvir with ribavirin led to an SVR12 of 92% (22 of 24) compared with an SVR12 of 84% (21 of 25) with 12 weeks of therapy. The cirrhotic group included only 6 patients with an SVR12 of 67% (2 of 3) and 100% (3 of 3) with 12 and 24 weeks, respectively.[23]

TREATMENT OF HEPATITIS C VIRUS GENOTYPE 5 AND 6 INFECTION

There are scarce data on the use of DAA on patients with HCV genotypes 5 and 6 infection. The AASLD/IDSA recommends the use of SOF/LDV for 12 weeks in treatment-naive patients.[3] A small open-label study addressed the use of 12 weeks of SOF/LDV in patients with HCV genotype 6 infection; 92% of the 25 patients were treatment naive and were primarily Asian (88%). The therapy resulted in an SVR12 of 96% (24 of 25).[24]

FUTURE THERAPY

Several other new DAA regimens are in clinical development and attempting to both optimize the duration of therapy and simplifying treatment. Sofosbuvir/GS-5816 is a combination of a nucleotide polymerase inhibitor and an NS5A inhibitor. Twelve weeks of therapy with sofosbuvir/GS-5816 in treatment-naive and noncirrhotic patients is associated with an SVR of 100% in genotype 1 and 2 infection, in addition to an SVR of 93% in genotype 3 infection. However, shorter duration of therapy of 8 weeks with sofosbuvir/GS-5816 resulted in lower SVRs of 90% and 88% in patients with HCV genotype 1 and 2 infection, respectively.[25]

The combination of grazoprevir and elbasvir with and without ribavirin therapy for 12 or 18 weeks was also assessed in the C-WORTHy trial (hepatitis C Worldwide genotype One Regimen Testing in the Hard to cure). One arm of the C-WORTHy trial involved 123 treatment-naive patients with cirrhosis with genotype 1 infection. The use of grazoprevir (an HCV NS3/4A protease inhibitor) with elbasvir (an NS5A inhibitor) alone or with addition of ribavirin resulted in comparable SVR12 of 90% (no ribavirin) to 95% (with ribavirin) with 12 weeks of therapy and 94% (no ribavirin) to 97% (with ribavirin) with 18 weeks of therapy. Patients with subgenotype 1b infection faired numerically better than patients with subgenotype 1a infection in the 12-week (100% vs 94%) and 18-week arms (98% vs 93%).[26] However, the difference was not statistically significant.

Shorter durations of therapy were also attempted using the combination of a nucleotide inhibitor (sofosbuvir) with a combination of NS3/4A and NS5A inhibitors (grazoprevir/elbasvir) in the C-SWIFT trial. The trial assessed the success of 4 versus 6 weeks of therapy in 61 HCV-1-infected treatment-naive noncirrhotic patients and 6 versus 8 weeks of therapy in 41 treatment-naive patients with cirrhosis. In the noncirrhotic group, the 6 weeks' therapy arm led to higher SVR (86.7%) than in the 4 weeks' therapy arm (38.7%). Longer duration of therapy also led to similar results in the 8-week arm (94.7%) than in the 6-week arm (80%). Subanalysis of the results revealed that patients with HCV-1a infection did not do as well as the patients with HCV-1b infection across all arms of the trial. The SVR4/8 in the noncirrhotic group of patients with HCV-1a infection was only seen in 9 of 26 patients (35%) in the 4-week arm and in 22 of 26 patients (85%) in the 6-week arm compared with 3 of 5 (60%) and 4 of 4 (100%), respectively, in patients with HCV-1b infection. In patients with cirrhosis treated for 6 or 8 weeks, 13 of 16 patients (81%) and 14 of 15 (93%) patients with HCV-1a infection achieved SVR4/8 compared with 3 of 4 (75%) and 4 of 4 (100%) in patients with HCV-1b infection, respectively.[27]

Hepatitis C genotype 3 is becoming the more challenging genotype to treat with the newer DAAs. There are emerging data showing promise in achieving SVR of more than 90% with the next generation of DAAs. The ALLY-3 clinical trial included 101 treatment-naive patients with HCV genotype 3 infection treated with 12 weeks of sofosbuvir and daclatasvir. This combination resulted in a 90.1% (91 of 101) SVR12. Subgroup analysis revealed an SVR12 of 97% (73 of 75) in the noncirrhotic group and a significantly reduced SVR12 of only 58% in the cirrhotic patients.[28] Sofosbuvir and GS-5816 with and without ribavirin has also been studied in ELECTRON-2, a phase 2 clinical trial. The trial included 104 treatment-naive noncirrhotic patients with HCV genotype 3 infection treated for only 8 weeks. Preliminary data report an SVR12 of 96% to 100% in patients receiving 100 mg of sofosbuvir/GS-5816 ± ribavirin.[29]

Clinical trials for the treatment of patients with HCV genotype 5 and 6 infection are ongoing. A pilot study of 12 weeks' combination therapy of SOF/LDV showed an SVR result of 96% in 24 of 25 patients with HCV genotype 6 infection. Of the 25 patients studied, 2 patients had cirrhosis and 2 were treatment experienced. However, the reported data were inclusive of the 2 patients with cirrhosis and the 2 treatment-experienced patients in the studied cohort of the 25 patients.[24]

SUMMARY

There have been major advances in the field of hepatitis C. Multiple ongoing clinical trials with various DAAs are demonstrating high efficacy combined with shorter duration of treatment and good tolerability. The success of these advancements allowed the elimination of interferon-based therapy for HCV infection. Future treatments for hepatitis C will consist of all oral regimens that combine classes of treatment that will result in pangenotypic coverage and shorter durations. There are numerous clinical trials with next-generation DAAs already showing promise in shortening therapy, with no impact on SVR.

REFERENCES

1. Lavanchy D. Evolving epidemiology of hepatitis C virus. Clin Microbiol Infect 2011;17:107–15.
2. Saleem J, Simmons B, Hill AM. Effects of sustained virological response (SVR) on the risk of liver transplant, hepatocellular carcinoma, death and re-infection: meta-analysis of 129 studies in 23,309 patients with hepatitis C infection. Hepatology 2014;60:24.
3. AASLD/IDSA/IAS–USA. Recommendations for testing, managing, and treating hepatitis C. Available at: http://www.hcvguidelines.org. Accessed April 24, 2014.
4. Gane EJ, Stedman CA, Hyland RH, et al. Nucleotide polymerase inhibitor sofosbuvir plus ribavirin for hepatitis C. N Engl J Med 2013;368:34–44.
5. Osinusi A, Meissner EG, Lee YJ, et al. Sofosbuvir and ribavirin for hepatitis C genotype 1 in patients with unfavorable treatment characteristics: a randomized clinical trial. JAMA 2013;310:804–11.
6. Lalezari J, Nelson D, Hyland R, et al. Once daily sofosbuvir plus ribavirin for 12 and 24 weeks in treatment-naive patients with HCV infection: the QUANTUM study. J Hepatol 2013;58:S346.
7. Afdhal N, Zeuzem S, Kwo P, et al. Ledipasvir and sofosbuvir for untreated HCV genotype 1 infection. N Engl J Med 2014;370:1889–98.
8. Kowdley KV, Gordon SC, Reddy KR, et al. Ledipasvir and sofosbuvir for 8 or 12 weeks for chronic HCV without cirrhosis. N Engl J Med 2014;370:1879–88.
9. Feld JJ, Kowdley KV, Coakley E, et al. Treatment of HCV with ABT-450/r-ombitasvir and dasabuvir with ribavirin. N Engl J Med 2014;370:1594–603.
10. Ferenci P, Bernstein D, Lalezari J, et al. ABT-450/r-ombitasvir and dasabuvir with or without ribavirin for HCV. N Engl J Med 2014;370:1983–92.
11. Lawitz E, Sulkowski MS, Ghalib R, et al. Simeprevir plus sofosbuvir, with or without ribavirin, to treat chronic infection with hepatitis C virus genotype 1 in non-responders to pegylated interferon and ribavirin and treatment-naive patients: the COSMOS randomised study. Lancet 2014;384:1756–65.

12. Jensen D, O'Leary J, Pockros P, et al. Safety and efficacy of sofosbuvir-containing regimens for hepatitis C: real-world experience in a diverse, longitudinal observational cohort. Hepatology 2014;60:55A.
13. Dieterich D, Bacon B, Flamm S, et al. Evaluation of sofosbuvir and simeprevir-based regimens in the TRIO network: academic and community treatment of a real-world, heterogeneous population. Hepatology 2014;60:55A.
14. Sulkowski MS, Gardiner DF, Rodriguez-Torres M, et al. Daclatasvir plus sofosbuvir for previously treated or untreated chronic HCV infection. N Engl J Med 2014; 370:211–21.
15. Lawitz E, Mangia A, Wyles D, et al. Sofosbuvir for previously untreated chronic hepatitis C infection. N Engl J Med 2013;368:1878–87.
16. Jacobson IM, Gordon SC, Kowdley KV, et al. Sofosbuvir for hepatitis C genotype 2 or 3 in patients without treatment options. N Engl J Med 2013;368:1867–77.
17. Zeuzem S, Dusheiko GM, Salupere R, et al. Sofosbuvir and ribavirin in HCV genotypes 2 and 3. N Engl J Med 2014;370:1993–2001.
18. Poordad F, Hezode C, Trinh R, et al. ABT-450/r-ombitasvir and dasabuvir with ribavirin for hepatitis C with cirrhosis. N Engl J Med 2014;370:1973–82.
19. European Association for the Study of the Liver. EASL recommendations on treatment of hepatitis C 2014. J Hepatol 2014;61:373–95.
20. Kapoor R, Kohli A, Sidhartan S, et al. All oral treatment for genotype 4 chronic hepatitis C infection with sofosbuvir and ledipasvir: interim results from the NIAID SYNERGY trial. Hepatology 2014;60:321A.
21. Pol S, Reddy RK, Baykal T, et al. Interferon-free regimens of ombitasvir and ABT-450/r with or without ribavirin in patients with HCV genotype 4 infection: PEARL-I study results. Hepatology 2014;60:1129A.
22. Ruane PJ, Ain D, Stryker R, et al. Sofosbuvir plus ribavirin for the treatment of chronic genotype 4 hepatitis C virus infection in patients of Egyptian ancestry. J Hepatol 2014;62(5):1040–6.
23. Esmat GE, Shiha G, Omar RF, et al. Sofosbuvir plus ribavirin in the treatment of Egyptian patients with chronic genotype 4 HCV infection. Hepatology 2014;60: 662A.
24. Gane EJ, Hyland RH, An D, et al. High efficacy of LDV/SOF regimens for 12 weeks for patients with HCV genotype 3 or 6 infection. Hepatology 2014;60:LB-11.
25. Tran TT, Morgan TR, Thuluvath PJ, et al. Safety and efficacy of treatment with sofosbuvir+GS-5816±ribavirin for 8 or 12 weeks in treatment naïve patients with genotype 1-6 HCV infection. Hepatology 2013;60S:58A.
26. Lawitz E, Gane E, Pearlman B, et al. Efficacy and safety of 12 weeks versus 18 weeks of treatment with grazoprevir (MK-5172) and elbasvir (MK-8742) with or without ribavirin for hepatitis C virus genotype 1 infection in previously untreated patients with cirrhosis and patients with previous null response with or without cirrhosis (C-WORTHY): a randomised, open-label phase 2 trial. Lancet 2014; 385(9973):1075–86.
27. Lawitz E, Poordad F, Gutierrez JA, et al. C-SWIFT: MK-5172 + MK-8742 + sofosbuvir in treatment-naive patients with hepatitis C virus genotype 1 infection, with and without cirrhosis, for durations of 4, 6, or 8 weeks. Hepatology 2014;60:LB-33.
28. Nelson DR, Cooper JN, Lalezari JP, et al. All-oral 12-week treatment with daclatasvir plus sofosbuvir in patients with hepatitis C virus genotype 3 infection: ALLY-3 phase 3 study. Hepatology 2015;61(4):1127–35.
29. Gane EJ, Hyland RH, Brainard DM, et al. Once daily sofosbuvir with GS-5816 for 8 weeks with or without ribavirin in patients with HCV genotype 3 without cirrhosis result in high rates of SVR12: the ELECTRON-2 study. Hepatology 2014;60:236A.

Direct-Acting Antiviral Agents

Regimens for the Interferon Failure Patient

Tatyana Kushner, MD, Vandana Khungar, MD, MSc*

KEYWORDS

- Hepatitis C • Direct-acting antivirals • Interferon • Treatment

KEY POINTS

- There are multiple reasons why patients failed interferon-containing treatments in the past, including intolerability to interferon, ineffective response to interferon, and relapse after treatment.
- With the emergence of new direct-acting antiviral agents (DAAs), there are multiple treatment options available to patients who have previously failed interferon-containing regimens.
- Hepatitis C genotype and severity of disease guide therapy choices in patients who have failed prior therapy.

INTRODUCTION

The treatment of hepatitis C has evolved dramatically since the historic days of exclusively interferon-containing therapy regimens and has continued to change rapidly since the initial introduction of direct-acting antiviral therapy in 2011. With the advent of multiple new treatment regimens, there are options for treatment now available to patients who previously failed interferon-containing therapy. Most of these regimens do not contain interferon, although in a few situations, interferon in combination with DAAs is still recommended for treatment. Most of the new drug regimens are highly effective and have minimal side effects, providing a dramatic improvement in tolerance and outcome of treatment on the course of the disease.

HISTORY OF INTERFERON-CONTAINING REGIMENS

Until recently, interferon-alfa combined with ribavirin was the mainstay of treatment of hepatitis C. In 1990, Hoofnagle and colleagues[1] demonstrated utilization of interferon

Dr T. Kushner is supported by a training grant NIH T32 (T32-DK007740-18). Dr V. Khungar has nothing to disclose.
Division of Gastroenterology and Hepatology, University of Pennsylvania, Philadelphia, PA, USA
* Corresponding author. 3400 Spruce Street, 2 Dulles, Philadelphia, PA 19104.
E-mail address: Vandana.Khungar@uphs.upenn.edu

alone for hepatitis C, which at the time was termed, *non-A, non-B hepatitis*. Interferon-alfa had been previously demonstrated to have a wide spectrum of antiviral activity against other viruses and was a "natural choice" as an initial therapeutic agent for hepatitis C. In this study, 10 patients were treated for a total of 12 months, and although 8 of 10 responded initially, only 10% of the study cohort demonstrated sustained virologic response (SVR) 1 year after treatment. In 2001, pegylated interferon was proposed as an alternative to interferon-alfa. The pegylated form of the drug has a covalently attached polyethylene glycol compound, which delays protein clearance and reduces immunogenicity, thereby resulting in a longer half-life of the drug, improved efficacy, and less frequent dosing. The properties of pegylated interferon allow for a decrease in adverse effects compared with standard interferon and improved patient adherence.[2] A randomized controlled trial comparing the pegylated form to interferon-alfa demonstrated increased SVR to up to 49% in the high-dose treatment group. The adverse effect profile was similar to interferon-alfa despite an increased SVR.[3]

Although ribavirin was initially proposed as potential therapeutic drug for hepatitis C in 1991[4] and used in combination with interferon-alfa in 1996 (improving SVR rates to 40%), it was not until 2001 that the first randomized controlled trial was performed by Manns and colleagues,[3] examining the synergistic effect of ribavirin with pegylated interferon in the treatment of hepatitis C. Patients were treated for 48 weeks, and SVR for patients treated with the combination of pegylated interferon and ribavirin increased to 54%, with SVR rates of approximately 80% in patients with genotypes 2 and 3. Subsequently, recommendations for the treatment of hepatitis C consisted of a combination of pegylated interferon and weight-based ribavirin for all patients with hepatitis C. Although these SVR rates were higher than previously reported, there was a significant amount of nonresponse to interferon-containing regimens in the real world.

Ten years later, the first generation of DAAs was discovered and integrated into clinical practice, in combination with pegylated interferon and ribavirin. Boceprevir and telaprevir were the first DAAs, both protease inhibitors, and were studied in the SPRINT-1 (Serine Protease Inhibitor-1), SPRINT-2 (Serine Protease Inhibitor-2), RESPOND-2 (Retreatment with HCV Serine Protease Inhibitor Boceprevir and Pegintron/Rebetrol 2), ILLUMINATE (Illustrating the Effects of Combination Therapy with Telaprevir), PROVE (Protease Inhibition for Viral Evaluation), and REALIZE (Retreatment of Telaprevir Based Regimen to Optimize Outcomes) studies.[5–9] These agents were approved in 2011 for the treatment of exclusively genotype 1 hepatitis C infection. Treatment with these agents in conjunction with pegylated interferon and ribavirin significantly increased SVR rates to up to 75% in treatment-naïve patients. Patients who were treated previously, however, had mixed results. Although prior treatment relapsers had response rates of 69% and 88%, prior partial responders had response rates of 40% and 59%, and prior null responders had response rates as low as 23% to 38%. There was, therefore, limited efficacy of these agents in patients who had been treated previously. In addition, these agents unfortunately were associated with severe side effects (severe anemia and rash), often worse than with pegylated interferon and ribavirin alone. They were associated with high pill burdens and restrictions on administering the medications with very high-fat meals and had low efficacy and safety in treatment-experienced patients. Most recently, several other DAAs have been developed and approved for use, thus broadening treatment options in patients who have previously failed interferon-containing regimens.

INTERFERON INTOLERABILITY

Prior to the discovery of DAAs for treatment of hepatitis C virus (HCV), treatment consisted of 24 to 48 week regimens of pegylated interferon and ribavirin. These treatments were associated with significant side effects and many patients had medical conditions that were contraindications to the use of interferon. Many patients, in particular those with severe psychiatric or autoimmune illness with concomitant chronic hepatitis C, were deemed unsuitable for these regimens as a result. Side effects of interferon-alfa and pegylated interferon-alfa were significant and more than 95% of patients on interferon reported at least 1 side effect in clinical trials,[10] although pegylated interferon was associated with slightly less frequent systemic side effects, such as fever, fatigue, and depression. The most frequent side effect reported was a flulike syndrome, including chills, fevers, joint pains, fatigue, and gastrointestinal distress. In addition, hematologic side effects, such as neutropenia and thrombocytopenia secondary to the myelosuppressive effect of interferon, occurred. Ribavirin, which is usually administered with interferon, further compounded hematologic abnormalities by causing a hemolytic anemia. Finally, severe psychiatric effects have been described with interferon use, from depression to suicidality, leading to significantly diminished quality of life, and many patients were either deemed too high risk for treatment or avoided treatment due to fear of these side effects. Other side effects of interferon include exacerbations of underlying autoimmune diseases (in particular, psoriasis); endocrinopathies, such as hypo- or hyperthyroidism; dermatologic side effects; and neurologic side effects, such as peripheral neuropathy. Some of these effects, such as dermatologic side effects, are exacerbated and more frequent when adding ribavirin. Thus, interferon-containing regimens were difficult for patients to tolerate and limited adherence, potentially contributing to treatment failure.[11]

INTERFERON FAILURE

Patients in whom interferon-containing regimens do not achieve durable SVR are considered to have failed interferon. Positive hepatitis C RNA testing at least 6 months after HCV therapy is concluded to confirm this failure. Prior to the current era of new DAAs, patients were categorized into groups of null responders, partial responders, and relapsers. Null responders were thought resistant to the effect of interferon, whereas partial responders or relapsers were thought to have a potentially correctable factor in treatment that could allow for a response.[12] Current treatment guidelines view these populations of patients similarly – whether patients previously did not respond, relapsed, or exhibited partial response, they generally qualify for the same regimens. With new DAAs available, retreatment of patients who previously failed interferon is recommended with predominantly interferon-free regimens, although certain patients still may benefit from interferon in conjunction with DAAs despite prior interferon failure.

Currently Recommended Treatment Regimens for Interferon Failure Patients: A Review of the Evidence and Current Guidelines

With the rapid development and Food and Drug Administration (FDA) approval of DAAs for the treatment of hepatitis C, guidelines for treatment of patients who have failed prior interferon-containing treatment have become available. Although many of these new treatment regimens are highly effective, cost-effectiveness of treatment of patients (who have previously been treated) will continue to be an ongoing debate, with the extremely high costs of newly emerging therapies limiting the ability to treat all patients with hepatitis C (**Tables 1–5** list cost data on available regimens). For instance, the cost of treatment regimens for genotype 1 hepatitis C ranges from $63,000 to $300,000, a significant cost burden, especially considering these patient have failed treatment previously and have potentially accrued previous costs from prior hepatitis C care.

Table 1
Estimated medication cost for treatment of genotype 1 chronic hepatitis C

Regimen and Duration of Therapy	Cost ($)
Ledipasvir/sofosbuvir × 8 wk	63,000
Ledipasvir/sofosbuvir × 12 wk	94,500
Ledipasvir/sofosbuvir × 24 wk	189,000
Ombitasvir/paritaprevir/ritonavir + dasabuvir ± ribavirin × 12 wk	84,000
Ombitasvir/paritaprevir/ritonavir + dasabuvir ± ribavirin × 24 wk	168,000
Sofosbuvir + simeprevir ± ribavirin × 12 wk	150,000
Sofosbuvir + simeprevir ± ribavirin × 24 wk	300,000

Cost data adapted from Hepatitis C Online. Available at: http://www.hepatitisc.uw.edu/.

Table 2
Estimated medication cost for treatment of genotype 2 chronic hepatitis C

Regimen and Duration of Therapy	Cost ($)
Sofosbuvir + ribavirin × 12 wk	85,000
Sofosbuvir + ribavirin × 16 wk	113,000
Sofosbuvir + ribavirin + pegylated interferon-alfa × 12 wk	97,000

Table 3
Estimated medication cost for treatment of genotype 3 chronic hepatitis C

Regimen and Duration of Therapy	Cost ($)
Sofosbuvir + ribavirin × 24 wk	169,000
Sofosbuvir + ribavirin + pegylated interferon-alfa × 12 wk	97,000

Table 4
Estimated medication cost for treatment of genotype 4 chronic hepatitis C

Regimen and Duration of Therapy	Cost ($)
Ledipasvir/sofosbuvir × 12 wk	94,500
Ombitasvir/paritaprevir/ritonavir + dasabuvir ± ribavirin × 12 wk	84,000
Sofosbuvir + ribavirin × 24 wk	169,000
Sofosbuvir + ribavirin + pegylated interferon × 12 wk	97,000
Sofosbuvir + simeprevir ± ribavirin × 12 wk	150,000

Table 5
Estimated medication cost for treatment of genotypes 5 and 6 chronic hepatitis C

Regimen and Duration of Therapy	Cost ($)
Sofosbuvir + ribavirin + pegylated interferon × 12 wk	97,000
Ledipasvir/sofosbuvir × 12 wk	94,500
Ribavirin + pegylated interferon × 48 wk	27,000

Nonetheless, up-to-date treatment guidelines have been made available integrating current therapies as they gain FDA approval, through the joint efforts of the American Association for the Study of Liver Diseases (AASLD), the Infectious Diseases Society of America, and the International Antiviral Society–USA, through evaluation of the current evidence of treatment and expert opinion, which are available on the www.hcvguidelines. org Web site. Current guidelines provide specific recommendations for patients who have failed prior treatment with pegylated interferon and ribavirin. Recommended treatment regimens are categorized by HCV genotype. Current treatment recommendations and outcomes of supporting clinical trials are summarized in **Tables 6–10**.

Table 6
Efficacy of regimens in genotype 1 hepatitis C virus treatment–experienced patients with and without cirrhosis

Regimen	Duration	Patient Population (Trial)	Sustained Virologic Response at Week 12 (%)	Patients
SOF + SIM	12 wk	F0-F2 null (COSMOS)	93	14
		F3-F4 (COSMOS)	100	7
SOF + SIM + RBV	12 wk	F0-F2 null (COSMOS)	96	27
		F3-F4 null (COSMOS)	93	15
LDV + SOF	12 wk	Noncirrhotic (ION-2)	95	87
		Cirrhotic (ION-2)	86	22
LDV + SOF	24 wk	Noncirrhotic (ION-2)	99	87
		Cirrhotic (ION-2)	100	22
LDV + SOF + RBV	12 wk	Noncirrhotic (ION-2)	100	89
		Cirrhotic (ION-2)	82	22
LDV + SOF + RBV	24 wk	Noncirrhotic (ION-2)	99	89
		Cirrhotic (ION-2)	100	22
3-D regimen + RBV	12 wk	Noncirrhotic (SAPPHIRE-II)		
		Prior relapse	95	86
		Prior partial response	100	65
		Prior null response	95	146
		Cirrhotic (TURQUOISE-II)		
		Prior relapse	97	29
		Prior partial response	94	18
		Prior null response	87	75
3-D regimen + RBV	24 wk	Cirrhotic (TURQUOISE-II)		
		Prior relapse	100	23
		Prior partial response	100	13
		Prior null response	95	62

Longer duration therapies of regimens (as opposed to 12-week regimens) shaded in gray.
Abbreviations: 3-D regimen, paritaprevir/ombitasvir/dasabuvir ± ribavirin; F0, no fibrosis; F1, mild fibrosis; F2, moderate fibrosis; F3, severe fibrosis; F4, cirrhosis; LDV, ledipasvir; PEG-IFN, pegylated interferon; RBV, ribavirin; SIM, simeprevir; SOF, sofosbuvir.

Table 7
Efficacy of regimens in genotype 2 hepatitis C virus treatment–experienced patients with and without cirrhosis

Regimen	Duration	Patient Population (Trial)	Sustained Virologic Response at Week 12 (%)	Patients
SOF + RBV	12 wk	Noncirrhotic (FUSION)	96	26
		Noncirrhotic (VALENCE)	94	32
		Cirrhotic (FUSION)	60	10
		Cirrhotic (VALENCE)	78	9
SOF + RBV	16 wk	Noncirrhotic (FUSION)	100	23
		Cirrhotic (FUSION)	78	9
SOF + RBV + PEG-IFN	12 wk	Noncirrhotic (LONESTAR-2)	93	14
		Cirrhotic (LONESTAR-2)	100	9

GENOTYPES 1A AND 1B TREATMENT RECOMMENDATIONS

Several clinical trials have demonstrated excellent outcomes in patients with hepatitis C genotype 1 who had been previously treated with interferon and did not initially achieve SVR (see **Table 6**). The COSMOS study (Combination of Simeprevir and Sofosbuvir in HCV genotype 1 infected patients), published in November 2014, investigated the use of simeprevir (an NS3/4A protease inhibitor) and sofosbuvir (an NS5B polymerase inhibitor), with or without ribavirin, as the first interferon-free treatment regimen.[13] The trial enrolled both treatment-naïve patients and nonresponders to pegylated interferon and ribavirin. SVR (sustained virologic response) at week 12 (SVR12) was achieved in 92% to 94% of patients, according to their fibrosis score; 2% of patients reported serious adverse events and 2% discontinued the trial due to adverse events. This therapy rapidly gained clinical popularity as the first interferon-free option for treatment of genotype 1 hepatitis C.

The ION-II trial published in April 2014 was a phase 3, randomized, open-label study involving patients with HCV genotype 1 who had been previously treated with pegylated interferon and ribavirin with or without a protease inhibitor.[14] Patients were randomly assigned to receive ledipasvir, an NS5A inhibitor, and sofosbuvir, a nucleotide polymerase inhibitor, in a once-daily fixed-dose combination tablet for 12 or 24 weeks, with or without ribavirin; 20% of the patients who received the treatment had cirrhosis. The SVR in all of the treatment groups was greater than 94%, with

Table 8
Efficacy of regimens in genotype 3 hepatitis C virus treatment–experienced patients with and without cirrhosis

Regimen	Duration	Patient Population (Trial)	Sustained Virologic Response at Week 12 (%)	Patients
SOF + RBV	12 wk	Noncirrhotic (FUSION)	37	38
		Cirrhotic (FUSION)	19	26
SOF + RBV	16 wk	Noncirrhotic (FUSION)	63	40
		Cirrhotic (FUSION)	61	23
SOF + RBV	24 wk	Noncirrhotic (VALENCE)	87	13
		Cirrhotic (VALENCE)	62	47
SOF + RBV + PEG-IFN	12 wk	Noncirrhotic and cirrhotic (LONESTAR-2)	83	12

Table 9
Efficacy of regimens in genotype 4 hepatitis C virus treatment–experienced patients with and without cirrhosis

Regimen	Duration	Patient Population (Trial)	Sustained Virologic Response at Week 12 (%)	Patients
LDV + SOF	12 wk	Cirrhotic/noncirrhotic (SYNERGY)	—	8
3-D regimen + RBV	12 wk	Noncirrhotic (PEARL)	100	41
SOF + RBV + PEG-IFN	12 wk	No study in treatment-experienced population[a]	—	—
SOF + RBV[21]	24 wk	Cirrhotic/noncirrhotic (AASLD 2014, Esmat et al)	96	27

[a] NEUTRINO study did show 96% SVR in 27 treatment-naïve patients.

99% SVR in each of the groups that received the treatment for 24 weeks. The results echoed those of ION-1, which involved patients who had not been previously treated. The most common adverse events included fatigue, headache, and nausea, and there were no subjects who discontinued therapy due to side effects. Thus, this therapy added to the arsenal of interferon-free treatment options for patients who had previously failed therapy.

The SAPPHIRE-II trial published in April 2014 enrolled patients with HCV genotype 1 who did not have cirrhosis who had been previously treated with pegylated interferon and ribavirin and had achieved a relapse, partial response, or null response.[15] Patients were randomly assigned to receive a new treatment, which consisted of paritaprevir, an NS3/4a protease inhibitor at a 150-mg once-daily dose, boosted with ritonavir, 100 mg daily; ombitasvir, an NS5a inhibitor at 25 mg daily; and dasabuvir, an NS5B inhibitor, at 250 mg twice daily; with ribavirin (1000 or 1200 mg daily) or matching placebo pills. In the 297 patients who were treated with the regimen, 96.3% of patients achieved SVR. This impressive SVR was compared with that of previously treated patients who had been secondarily treated with telaprevir, who only achieved an SVR of 65%. SVR ranged from 95.2% in prior null responders to 100% in patients with a prior partial response. The most common adverse events with this treatment regimen were headache and fatigue, with no moderate or severe adverse events reported. Similar to the ION trials, these results were almost identical to the results of SAPPHIRE-1, which enrolled patients who had not been treated previously. This treatment regimen became the third all-oral regimen to be available for clinical use.

Table 10
Efficacy of regimens in genotypes 5 and 6 hepatitis C virus treatment–experienced patients with and without cirrhosis

Regimen	Duration	Patient Population (Trial)
SOF + RBV + PEG-IFN	12 wk	No trial in treatment-experienced patients[a]
PEG-IFN + RBV	48 wk	—
LDV + SOF	12 wk	Genotype 6 only[b]

[a] NEUTRINO study did show 100% SVR in 7 treatment-naïve patients.
[b] Several studies have shown safety and efficacy of this regimen in genotype 6 although data are limited.

The UNITY 2 study had an arm of patients with HCV genotype 1 who had been previously treated to evaluate the safety and efficacy of a combined regimen, including daclatasvir, an NS5a inhibitor; asunaprevir, an NS3 protease inhibitor; and BMS-791325, a non-nucleoside NS5B inhibitor with or without ribavirin[16]; 96% of all patients who received the combination with ribavirin achieved SVR and 90% of those who received the combination without ribavirin achieved SVR. This therapy is currently not available in the United States.

Therefore, the COSMOS, ION-II, and SAPPHIRE-II studies led to the development of the current guidelines for the treatment of genotype 1 disease. Current guidelines state that for patients with HCV genotype 1a or genotype 1b infection without cirrhosis who have failed prior treatments, there are currently 3 available regimens that are equally effective. There is a class I, level A recommendation for treatment with a daily fixed-dose combination of ledipasvir/sofosbuvir, now marketed as Harvoni (Gilead, Foster City, CA), or a daily fixed-dose combination of paritaprevir/ritonavir/ombitasvir plus twice-daily dasabuvir along with weight-based ribavirin, called the 3-D regimen, and recently approved by the FDA and marketed as the Viekira Pak. In addition there is a class IIa, level B recommendation for the use of sofosbuvir and simeprevir with or without weight-based ribavirin, marketed as Sovaldi and Olysio, which are currently less frequently used in clinical practice.

Different treatment guidelines apply to patients with HCV genotype 1 with cirrhosis. The SIRIUS trial evaluated prior nonresponders with cirrhosis and randomized them to ledipasvir/sofosbuvir with ribavirin for 12 weeks or without ribavirin for 24 weeks and found similarly high SVR rates of above 95% in both study groups. The study was presented at the AASLD conference in 2014. Thus, current guidelines recommend that in a patient with HCV genotype 1a or 1b with compensated cirrhosis who previously failed interferon-containing regimens, the duration of treatment with ledipasvir/sofosbuvir should be extended to 24 weeks or maintained at 12 weeks if used in combination with weight-based ribavirin (the less preferred option due to side effects).

The TURQUOISE-II study addressed the use of paritaprevir/ritonavir/ombitasvir plus dasubavir for 12 or 24 weeks in treatment experienced patients with cirrhosis.[17] This study found higher SVR rates in patients treated with 24 weeks versus 12 weeks of therapy and higher response rates in patients with genotype 1b versus 1a HCV. Thus, current guidelines support the combination of paritaprevir/ritonavir/ombitasvir plus twice-daily dasabuvir (as described previously) with weight-based ribavirin for 24 weeks if the patient has genotype 1a disease but not in 1b disease. Similar to the recommendation in noncirrhotic patients, there is a class IIa, level B recommendation to use sofosbuvir plus simeprevir with or without weight-based ribavirin for 24 weeks in this patient group based on results from the COSMOS study.

In patients without advanced fibrosis in whom therapy regimens with sofosbuvir have failed in the past, guidelines at this time recommend deferring treatment until new therapies become available given the lack of clinical data on treatment. In patients who have failed prior sofosbuvir-containing treatment with advanced fibrosis, however, current recommendations are to use a daily fixed-dose combination of ledipasvir/sofosbuvir with or without weight-based ribavirin for the longer duration of 24 weeks, which is a class IIa, level C recommendation, because these patients cannot wait for new treatments to become available.

For patients with genotype 1 infection who have failed prior pegylated interferon, ribavirin, and protease inhibitor regimens, there is evidence to suggest that resistance may occur to other protease inhibitors, and thus retreatment with protease inhibitors is not recommended. Treatment with ledipasvir/sofosbuvir for 12 weeks, however, is recommended in this scenario. In patients with cirrhosis who have failed a protease-containing regimen, the duration of treatment recommended with these agents is lengthened to 24 weeks or remains 12 weeks if ribavirin is added. In this patient population, in addition to not retreating with other protease inhibitors, current guidelines strongly recommend also not treating again with any interferon-containing regimen, including with first- and second-generation DAAs in combination with interferon.

GENOTYPES 2 AND 3 TREATMENT RECOMMENDATIONS

In patients with genotype 2 hepatitis C who have previously failed therapy with pegylated interferon and ribavirin, the current recommended regimen is sofosbuvir and ribavirin. The FUSION study included a randomized controlled trial with patients who had previously not responded to interferon therapy for 12 or 16 weeks.[18] The response rate was 50% with 12 weeks of treatment and 73% with 16 weeks of treatment, although subsequent studies, including the VALENCE study, reported equal efficacy with a 12-week duration of treatment.[19] Therefore, the current recommended treatment is daily sofosbuvir and weight-based ribavirin for 12 to 16 weeks. This patient population is among the few treatment-failure patient groups in which there is a class IIa, level B recommendation to use sofosbuvir/ribavirin in combination with pegylated interferon if patients are eligible to receive interferon, based on the results of the LONESTAR-2 trial.[20]

In patients with genotype 3 infection, treatment with sofosbuvir/ribavirin is also recommended, although duration of treatment is longer, with 24 weeks recommended, based on results of the VALENCE trial. The same alternative regimen consisting of pegylated interferon and ribavirin, as was recommended for treatment of patients with genotype 2, also has a class IIa, level B recommendation for genotype 3.

GENOTYPES 4, 5, AND 6 TREATMENT RECOMMENDATIONS

Unlike for genotypes 1, 2, and 3 disease, the data guiding treatment options in patients with genotypes 4, 5, and 6 disease in whom prior treatment with interferon has failed are somewhat limited. The phase 2b PEARL-1 study evaluated the efficacy of paritaprevir/ritonavir/ombitasvir with or without ribavirin in patients with genotype 4 and included patients who had previously failed therapy. SVR12 was achieved in 100% of patients (although none of these patients was cirrhotic). In addition, sofosbuvir with pegylated interferon and ribavirin was investigated in genotype 4 patients in the NEUTRINO trial whereas ledipasvir/sofosbuvir was investigated in the SYNERGY trial, with similarly high SVR rates. Finally, Esmat and colleagues presented a study at AASLD in 2014 examining sofosbuvir/ribavirin (without interferon) and found 87% SVR12 in patients treated for 24 weeks compared with 40% in those treated for 12 weeks.[21] Therefore, in patients with genotype 4 infection, in whom prior treatment with pegylated interferon and ribavirin have failed, there are 4 possible treatment options. Three of these consist of 12-week regimens, namely ledipasvir/sofosbuvir, paritaprevir/ritonavir/ombitasvir/ribavirin, and sofosbuvir/ribavirin with retreatment with pegylated interferon. A 24-week course with sofosbuvir/ribavirin is also an alternative course of treatment.

For genotype 5–infected patients in whom prior treatment has failed, the only treatment options available involve the use of interferon, with either a 12-week course of sofosbuvir, with pegylated interferon and ribavirin, or a 48-week course of ribavirin and pegylated interferon alone.

For genotype 6 infection, fortunately, ledipasvir has been found effective.[22,23] Therefore, for genotype 6 infection, a 12-week treatment with ledipasvir/sofosbuvir is recommended, with an alternative of a 12-week course of sofosbuvir and ribavirin with weekly interferon for 12 weeks, shown effective in the NEUTRINO trial in a small number of patients with genotype 6.[24]

SUMMARY

The rapidly evolving treatment options for hepatitis C in patients who have failed prior therapy with interferon have dramatically improved outcomes and will likely continue to do so in future years. Patients who have failed prior therapy should be encouraged to seek treatment now that effective therapies with minimal side effects are available. Although outcomes with treatment of patients with genotype 1 disease have been excellent, retreatment of patients with genotype 3 disease remains a problem, because there is still clearly a role for interferon despite prior interferon failure, and SVR rates are not as high as they are for genotype 1. In addition, data are limited in patients who have genotypes 4, 5, and 6 who have been previously treated. Further studies of real-world outcomes with newer regimens are necessary to determine long-term outcomes in patients on these therapies. Nonetheless, the ability to treat and cure patients with hepatitis C who have previously not responded to treatment will change the course of the disease for many years to come.

REFERENCES

1. Hoofnagle JH, Mullen KD, Jones DB, et al. Treatment of chronic non-A, non-B hepatitis with recombinant human alpha interferon. A preliminary report. N Engl J Med 1986;315:1575–8.
2. Degasperi E, Vigano M, Aghemo A, et al. PegIFN-alpha2a for the treatment of chronic hepatitis B and C: a 10-year history. Expert Rev Anti Infect Ther 2013; 11:459–74.
3. Manns MP, McHutchison JG, Gordon SC, et al. Peginterferon alfa-2b plus ribavirin compared with interferon alfa-2b plus ribavirin for initial treatment of chronic hepatitis C: a randomised trial. Lancet 2001;358:958–65.
4. Reichard O, Andersson J, Schvarcz R, et al. Ribavirin treatment for chronic hepatitis C. Lancet 1991;337:1058–61.
5. Kwo PY, Lawitz EJ, McCone J, et al. Efficacy of boceprevir, an NS3 protease inhibitor, in combination with peginterferon alfa-2b and ribavirin in treatment-naive patients with genotype 1 hepatitis C infection (SPRINT-1): an open-label, randomised, multicentre phase 2 trial. Lancet 2010;376:705–16.
6. Poordad F, McCone J Jr, Bacon BR, et al. Boceprevir for untreated chronic HCV genotype 1 infection. N Engl J Med 2011;364:1195–206.
7. Welch NM, Jensen DM. Pegylated interferon based therapy with second-wave direct-acting antivirals in genotype 1 chronic hepatitis C. Liver Int 2015; 35(Suppl 1):11–7.
8. Zeuzem S, Andreone P, Pol S, et al. Telaprevir for retreatment of HCV infection. N Engl J Med 2011;364:2417–28.
9. McHutchison JG, Everson GT, Gordon SC, et al. Telaprevir with peginterferon and ribavirin for chronic HCV genotype 1 infection. N Engl J Med 2009;360:1827–38.
10. Negro F. Adverse effects of drugs in the treatment of viral hepatitis. Best Pract Res Clin Gastroenterol 2010;24:183–92.
11. Younossi Z, Henry L. Systematic review: patient-reported outcomes in chronic hepatitis C - the impact of liver disease and new treatment regimens. Aliment Pharmacol Ther 2015;41:497–520.

12. Shiffman ML. Chronic hepatitis C: treatment of pegylated interferon/ribavirin non-responders. Curr Gastroenterol Rep 2006;8:46–52.
13. Lawitz E, Sulkowski MS, Ghalib R, et al. Simeprevir plus sofosbuvir, with or without ribavirin, to treat chronic infection with hepatitis C virus genotype 1 in non-responders to pegylated interferon and ribavirin and treatment-naive patients: the COSMOS randomised study. Lancet 2014;384:1756–65.
14. Afdhal N, Zeuzem S, Kwo P, et al. Ledipasvir and sofosbuvir for untreated HCV genotype 1 infection. N Engl J Med 2014;370:1889–98.
15. Feld JJ, Kowdley KV, Coakley E, et al. Treatment of HCV with ABT-450/r-ombitasvir and dasabuvir with ribavirin. N Engl J Med 2014;370:1594–603.
16. Everson GT, Sims KD, Rodriguez-Torres M, et al. Efficacy of an interferon- and ribavirin-free regimen of daclatasvir, asunaprevir, and BMS-791325 in treatment-naive patients with HCV genotype 1 infection. Gastroenterology 2014;146:420–9.
17. Poordad F, Hezode C, Trinh R, et al. ABT-450/r-ombitasvir and dasabuvir with ribavirin for hepatitis C with cirrhosis. N Engl J Med 2014;370:1973–82.
18. Jacobson IM, Gordon SC, Kowdley KV, et al. Sofosbuvir for hepatitis C genotype 2 or 3 in patients without treatment options. N Engl J Med 2013;368:1867–77.
19. Zeuzem S, Dusheiko GM, Salupere R, et al. Sofosbuvir and ribavirin in HCV genotypes 2 and 3. N Engl J Med 2014;370:1993–2001.
20. Lawitz E, Poordad FF, Pang PS, et al. Sofosbuvir and ledipasvir fixed-dose combination with and without ribavirin in treatment-naive and previously treated patients with genotype 1 hepatitis C virus infection (LONESTAR): an open-label, randomised, phase 2 trial. Lancet 2014;383:515–23.
21. Doss W, Shiha G, Hassany M, et al. Sofosbuvir plus ribavirin for treating Egyptian patients with hepatitis C genotype 4. J Hepatol 2015. [Epub ahead of print].
22. Wong KA, Worth A, Martin R, et al. Characterization of Hepatitis C virus resistance from a multiple-dose clinical trial of the novel NS5A inhibitor GS-5885. Antimicrob Agents Chemother 2013;57:6333–40.
23. Kohler JJ, Nettles JH, Amblard F, et al. Approaches to hepatitis C treatment and cure using NS5A inhibitors. Infect Drug Resist 2014;7:41–56.
24. Lawitz E, Mangia A, Wyles D, et al. Sofosbuvir for previously untreated chronic hepatitis C infection. N Engl J Med 2013;368:1878–87.

Mechanisms of Virologic Failure with Direct-Acting Antivirals in Hepatitis C and Strategies for Retreatment

Vanessa Costilla, MD[a], Neha Mathur, MD[a], Julio A. Gutierrez, MD, MS[b],*

KEYWORDS

- Hepatitis C • Retreatment • Genotype 1 • Direct-acting antivirals (DAAs)
- Resistance-associated variants (RAVs) • Protease inhibitor
- RNA-polymerase inhibitor • NS5A inhibitor

KEY POINTS

- Pharmacologic, viral and host factors all may contribute to treatment failure in the DAA era.
- The presence of Resistance Associated Variants (RAVs) may impact therapy during retreatment with DAAs. Commercial testing is available.
- Salvage therapy in DAA experienced patients is still an area of emerging research, and each patient's treatment plan should be individualized.

INTRODUCTION

The most effective therapies against hepatitis C use small molecules known as direct-acting antivirals (DAAs).[1] Up to 170 million people worldwide may be infected with the hepatitis C virus (HCV),[2] and virologic failure to DAAs will likely be of significant public health concern in the future. Clinical trials have shown high rates of cure, determined by eradication of the virus at 12 weeks after treatment (known as sustained virologic response 12 [SVR12]). Real-world data suggest that virologic failure will occur more commonly. The reason for DAA virologic failure in an individual depends on the

Dr J.A. Gutierrez serves on scientific advisory boards or has received research grants from Gilead and Abbvie. He is a speaker for Janssen Therapeutics and Abbvie. Drs V. Costilla and N. Mathur have nothing to disclose.
[a] Department of Hepatology, University of Texas Health Science Center at San Antonio, 7703 Floyd Curl Drive, San Antonio, TX 78229, USA; [b] Department of Hepatology, The Texas Liver Institute, University of Texas Health Science Center at San Antonio, 607 Camden, San Antonio, TX 78215, USA
* Corresponding author.
E-mail address: Gutierrezj8@uthscsa.edu

Clin Liver Dis 19 (2015) 641–656
http://dx.doi.org/10.1016/j.cld.2015.06.005
1089-3261/15/$ – see front matter © 2015 Elsevier Inc. All rights reserved.

efficacy of the regimen chosen but may be impacted by pharmacokinetics, poor patient adherence, poor tolerability, viral resistance, and host factors. Strategies to avoid virologic failure and utilization of salvage therapy are of increasing importance.

In 2011, the first DAAs approved for genotype 1–infected patients were the protease inhibitors (PIs), telaprevir and boceprevir. These drugs required coadministration with interferon/ribavirin (RBV) and were associated with high rates of treatment discontinuation secondary to adverse events and viral breakthrough, along with relapse after the end of treatment. Although little data exist on the total number of patients who have experienced virologic failure after DAA therapy is unknown, data from real-world SVR12 reports may guide estimates. More than 100,000 prescriptions of telaprevir and boceprevir were issued worldwide. These agents were approved for the treatment of genotype 1–infected patients only. Real-world data suggest that 36% to 49% of individuals failed therapy.[3,4] Those treated with these agents may have PI resistance-associated variants (RAVs) that could complicate retreatment with a PI-based therapy.

In 2013, 2 additional DAAs, sofosbuvir (SOF) and simeprevir (SIM), were approved. Since the availability of SOF and SIM, thousands of prescriptions for DAAs have been initiated (**Fig. 1**). In part, this initial wave of therapy was driven by the study known as COSMOS (Combination Of SiMeprevir and sOfosbuvir in HCV genotype 1 infected patientS),[5] which revealed good efficacy and tolerability of the combination of SOF and SIM in genotype 1, albeit in small numbers. At the moment, 2 other interferon (IFN)-free regimens (paritaprevir/ritonavir [r]/ombitasvir/dasabuvir and SOF/ledipasvir [LDV]) are also commercially available in the United States.

Despite the enthusiasm for all-oral, interferon-free therapy, higher rates of virologic failure were seen in early evaluation of real-world data. The mechanism of relapse after therapy with DAAs is still poorly understood. Retreatment with SOF with IFN and/or RBV in previous failures may result in SVR12 based on initial studies. In genotype 1–infected individuals with prior SOF failure, SVR12 can also be achieved with SOF by adding LDV with or without RBV. Whether other regimens, such as paritaprevir/r/ombitasvir/dasabuvir, or other agents in the DAA pipeline can be used for retreatment of SOF failures still has not been studied. Other regimens that use 3 potent DAAs are forthcoming. Triplet regimens with nonoverlapping mechanisms are expected to have high efficacy because the impact of individual RAVs are diminished. Data regarding

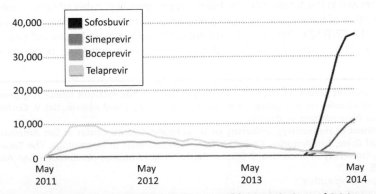

Fig. 1. Rising DAA use in the United States. The monthly prescriptions of DAAs reported to the Intercontinental Marketing Services (IMS) are shown from May 2011 to May 2014. (*Data from* Harbingers of change in healthcare: implications for the role and use of medicines. IMS (Danbury, CT); 2014.)

retreatment of PI failures with next-generation PIs are lacking, although resistance testing may guide the clinician. Novel nucleotide analogues, such as MK-3682 (formerly IDX-437) or ACH-3422, may play roles in salvage therapy; but no studies have been conducted at the time of this publication. Other agents with efficacy in genotype 2 and 3, such as daclatasvir, may also be used in retreatment as they become commercially available.

MECHANISMS OF DIRECT-ACTING ANTIVIRAL DRUGS

In-depth understanding of the HCV life cycle and genomics has facilitated the development of novel target therapeutics. HCV is an RNA virus that uses the host ribosome as the translational machinery to produce a polyprotein, which is then cleaved into structural (core, E1, and E2) and nonstructural (P7, NS2, NS3/NS4A, NS4B, NS5A, and NS5B) proteins. Genetic heterogeneity is significant in HCV because of the lack of proofreading on the part of the RNA-dependent RNA polymerase (NS5B).

Elaboration of key tools and models, including infectious cell clones, the replicons, complete cell culture systems, and genetically humanized mice where the HCV life cycle can be recapitulated in vivo, has accelerated drug development. Along with these major breakthroughs, the understanding of the 3-dimensional structures of the HCV proteins also greatly facilitated the target of DAAs. There are currently 4 classes of DAA drugs that target specific proteins within the HCV replication cycle. These classes include nonstructural proteins 3/4A (NS3/4A) PIs, NS5A inhibitors, NS5B nucleoside polymerase inhibitors (NPI), and NS5B non-nucleoside polymerase inhibitors (NNPIs). In some cases, patients may have been exposed to multiple agents over time (**Table 1**).

Protease Inhibitors

NS3/4A PIs disrupt post-translation processing and replication of HCV.[1] NS3 possesses the proteolytic activity, whereas NS4 acts as cofactor. PIs block the NS3 catalytic site or NS3/NS4 binding.[1] First-generation PIs include telaprevir and boceprevir. Telaprevir and boceprevir are substrates of CYP3A4 (cytochrome P) and are primarily metabolized in the liver. Because of their low barriers to resistance and toxicities, they have fallen out of favor and are no longer available in the United States.

Second-wave and next-generation PIs include SIM and paritaprevir. SIM is metabolized primarily in the liver and intestine and is also a CYP3A4 substrate. Paritaprevir is

Table 1
Potential sources of DAA-experienced patients

Regimen	DAAs
PEG-IFN/RBV + PI	Telaprevir, boceprevir, SIM
PEG-IFN/RBV or RBV + SOF	SOF
Sequential DAA failure[a]	First DAA therapy: telaprevir, boceprevir Second DAA therapy: SOF or SOF/LDV
Concurrent 2 class failure	SOF/SIM or SOF/LDV
Concurrent 3 class failure	Paritaprevir/r/ombitasvir/dasabuvir.

Because patients from clinical trials are small in number, those who received agents as part of clinical trials that have not been FDA approved are not included. Retreatment with PIs is currently not recommended, and there should be few patients in this scenario.

Abbreviation: PEG, pegylated.
[a] SIM was not included as possible mono-DAA failure because there was little uptake with PEG-IFN/RBV.

metabolized by CYP3A4 and CYP2D6 to a lesser extent. Paritaprevir is only available in fixed-dose combination with ombitasvir and ritonavir.

NS5A Inhibitors

NS5A acts in the organization of the replication complex, in regulating replication, and in the assembly of the viral particle released from the host cell.[1] However, the precise mechanisms through which these are achieved remain unknown. LDV and ombitasvir are both NS5A inhibitors approved in the United States. Daclatasvir is not yet available in the United States during the preparation of this article but is approved in Europe.

LDV is only available in fixed-dosed combination with sofosbuvir. LDV undergoes slow oxidative metabolism via an unknown mechanism. Ombitasvir is only available in fixed-dose combination with paritaprevir, ritonavir, and dasabuvir, which are collectively sold as Viekira Pak. Ombitasvir is metabolized by amide hydrolysis and oxidative metabolism.

NS5B Non-nucleoside Polymerase Inhibitors

NS5B is an RNA-dependent RNA polymerase essential for viral replication through its involvement in post-translational processing. NS5B has a catalytic site for nucleoside binding and 4 other sites where a non-nucleoside compound may bind, resulting in allosteric alteration.[1]

NNPIs target the 4 sites that result in allosteric alteration. NNPIs are developed to be genotype specific, depending on which of the 4 allosteric sites are targeted. Dasabuvir is a genotype 1–specific NNPI approved for use with ombitasvir, paritaprevir, and ritonavir, although is formulated separately from the other agents. Dasabuvir is metabolized by CYP2C8, and to a lesser extent CYP3A.

NS5B Nucleoside Polymerase Inhibitors

NS5B NPIs target the catalytic site and result in chain termination during RNA replication of the viral genome. NPIs have broad efficacy across all genotypes and a high barrier to resistance. SOF is the first, and only, available NPI at this time. It is metabolized by the liver to form the pharmacologically active agent.

POTENTIAL FAILURE POPULATIONS
Mono–Direct-Acting Antiviral Therapy with Protease Inhibitor

Boceprevir and telaprevir were first generation PIs used in combination with pegylated-IFN (PEG-IFN) and RBV for the treatment of HCV genotype 1. The efficacy of these medications against HCV in treatment-naïve and experienced patients was described in 2011.[6–9] In noncirrhotic treatment-naïve patients, boceprevir demonstrated an SVR of 63% to 66%,[10] whereas, in a separate study, patients treated with telaprevir achieved an SVR of 75%.[8] Several baseline host and viral factors predicted the likelihood of SVR with both agents.

Since the approval of telaprevir and boceprevir for the treatment of HCV genotype 1, several studies have reported the real-world success of these medications. In a managed care, private setting, SVR was achieved in 55% of all patients, which included those with cirrhosis and those who had prior relapse or a null response to PEG-IFN and RBV alone. The overall SVR for those treated with telaprevir was 56% and 53% for those treated with boceprevir.[11] In a Veterans Affairs population, SVR was achieved in 51.5% of patients, which included those with cirrhosis and a prior relapse or a null response to PEG-IFN and RBV.[12] Those who had relapsed after treatment with PEG-IFN/RBV, had the highest overall success with an SVR of

64%. Unfortunately, only 34% to 35% of patients who started therapy with either boceprevir or telaprevir were able to complete the full 48 weeks of treatment.[12]

Those with advanced hepatic fibrosis and prior treatment experience fared poorly with boceprevir and telaprevir, even in rigorous studies. The CUPIC (Compassionate Use of Protease Inhibitors in Viral C Cirrhosis) study evaluated the effectiveness of telaprevir or boceprevir in conjunction with PEG-IFN/RBV in treatment-experienced patients with HCV genotype 1 and cirrhosis. Among the patients who received telaprevir, the overall SVR rate was 52%. Patients who were prior null responders had the lowest rates of SVR (19%).[13] Among the boceprevir recipients, 43% achieved SVR12. No patients (0 of 10) who were prior null responders were successfully treated with the regimen.[13] Another study of treatment-experienced patients reported an SVR of 59.8% in those treated with either telaprevir or boceprevir. Telaprevir-treated patients had a higher SVR of 65.9% compared with 44.0% of boceprevir-treated patients.[14]

SIM use is discussed only in combination with SOF because few clinicians used this agent as it was initially approved with PEG-IFN/RBV.[15,16]

Mono-Sofosbuvir Failures

Initially, SOF was approved in combination with PEG-IFN/RBV for genotype 1–infected patients or with RBV alone for non–genotype 1 patients. The NEUTRINO study evaluated the effectiveness of SOF in conjunction with PEG-IFN and RBV in patients with HCV genotype 1 with and without cirrhosis. In patients without cirrhosis, 92% achieved SVR12, whereas in those patients with cirrhosis, only 80% achieved SVR12.[17]

Early data presented at the American Association for the Study of Liver Diseases (AASLD) 2014 meeting from HCV-TARGET, an international consortium of investigators conducting a longitudinal observational study of HCV therapy with DAA agents, reported an SVR4 of 85% overall in patients with genotype 1 treated with SOF plus PEG-IFN/RBV. The SVR4 was lower in patients with cirrhosis (70%).[18] Patients with genotype 2 treated with 12 weeks of SOF/RBV had an overall SVR4 of 90%.

The TRIO Network collects prescription data from US academic and community medical centers and focuses on patients taking 12-week regimens of PEG-IFN/RBV plus SOF, SOF plus SIM with or without RBV, and SOF plus RBV alone. They reported overall SVR12 in patients with genotype 1 of 78% with PEG-IFN/RBV plus SOF.[19] Patients with genotype 2 treated with SOF/RBV had an overall SVR12 of 90%.

All Oral Treatment Failures

The COSMOS study evaluated the efficacy of SIM and SOF with/without RBV in patients with HCV genotype 1 who were treatment-naïve and experienced, including those with cirrhosis. SVR12 was achieved in 92% of patients in cohort 1 (previous nonresponders with METAVIR scores F0-F2) and in 94% of patients in cohort 2 (previous nonresponders and treatment-naïve patients with METAVIR scores F3-F4).[5] Based on these data, many clinicians began using this combination for 12 weeks with or without RBV for patients with HCV infected with genotype 1.

Data from HCV-TARGET report SVR4 in 86% of patients receiving SOF/SIM and 87% of those treated with SOF/SIM/RBV overall in those treated with SIM and SOF with/without RBV. Noncirrhotic patients and those with genotype 1b had higher SVR4 rates.[18] HCV-TARGET reported SVR4 of 81% for those who were prior PI failures.

Data from the TRIO Network reported SVR12 in patients with genotype 1 treated with SOF/SIM/with/without RBV. Noncirrhotic patients were more likely to be cured with this regimen (87%) compared with 76% of cirrhotic patients.[19]

Real-world data will likely soon be available regarding the efficacy of 2 other Food and Drug Administration (FDA)–approved regimens for genotype 1, SOF/LDV and paritaprevir/r/ombitasvir/dasabuvir, in the next year.

MECHANISM OF NONRESPONSE TO ANTIVIRAL

The factors associated with nonresponse to IFN therapy were a major topic of research during the last 2 decades. Race, comorbidities, interleukin 28B (IL28B) status, viral genotype/subtype, and degree of liver fibrosis emerged as major factors. When patients fail potent DAA regimens, the reasons for failure seem distinct from the IFN era, although some may retain some importance as clinicians begin to report their experiences (**Table 2**). Exploring these viral and host factors is vital to achieving improved cure rates and to identify nonresponders to improve cost-effectiveness of these therapies.[20]

Viral Factors

The RAVs of hepatitis C have been attributed to a high viral replication rate, high error rate of viral RNA-dependent RNA polymerase, and lack of overlapping reading frames in the hepatitis C nonstructural region.[20] The above-mentioned replicative errors lead to numerous variants known as HCV-quasispecies.[21] During HCV infection, the wild-type of virus predominates but when several isolates in the HCV-quasispecies can undergo mutations and then confer resistance to DAAs by directly or indirectly effects.[21] These mutations are the naturally occurring RAVs also known as HCV polymorphisms. It is also been known that SVRs vary by subtype of genotype 1, showing better SVR in genotype 1b than genotype 1a. This variation is attributed to lower genetic barriers to resistant variants at key sites on HCV NS3 protease in patients with genotype 1a compared with patients with 1b.[22]

For the first wave of NS3 PIs, telaprevir and boceprevir, the drug resistance variants have been identified by genotype 1a and 1b (**Table 3**). For telaprevir genotype 1a, the resistant variants are V36M, R155K, and V36M plus R155K.[22] For genotype 1b, the resistant variants include V36A, T54A/S, and A 156S/T/V.[22] For boceprevir genotype 1a, V36M, T54S, and R155K are the resistant variants; for genotype 1b

Table 2 Factors possibly affecting SVR12 in the DAA era	
Pharmacologic	Potency of drug Drug delivery and metabolism Drug-drug interactions Number of DAAs (dual vs triplet therapy)
Viral	Genotype/subtype RAVs Prior DAA experience
Host	IL28B status Prior IFN experience Degree of liver fibrosis Portal hypertension Portosystemic shunts Drug misuse/compliance Immune function

The impact of pharmacologic, viral, and host factors are still an era of evolving research; however, those listed in this table may be expected to impact virologic failure.

Table 3
NS3/4A in vitro RAVs

	Genotype 1a							Genotype 1b						
	V36M/A	T54S/A	Q80K	S122R/G	R155K	R155G	D168V/E/A	V36M/A	T54A/S	Q80R	S122A	R155Q	A156T/G	D168V/E/A
Boceprevir	+	+	−	−	+	−	−	+	+	−	−	−	+	−
Telaprevir	+	+	−	−	+	+	−	+	+	−	−	−	+	−
SIM	−	−	+	+	+	−	+	−	−	−	+	+	−	+
Paritaprevir	−	−	−	−	+	+	+	−	−	−	−	−	−	+
Grazoprevir	−	−	−	−	−	−	+	−	−	−	−	−	+	+

Common genotype 1a and 1b RAVs are shown here for approved and soon-to-be approved PIs.
Data from Refs.[22–24]

they are T54A/S, V55A, A156S, and I/V170A.[22] These RAVs have impaired production of the virus and viral proteins, and others increase replicative fitness of the virus.

For second-wave NS3 PIs, including SIM and paritaprevir, the main resistant variant is R155K in patients with genotype 1a; D168 A/V/E/T is noted in both genotype 1a and 1b. There is cross-resistance for R155K among first- and second-generation PIs in genotype 1a and A156 T/V for genotype 1b. Q80K polymorphism is common (prevalence 30%–40%) in genotype 1a showing resistance to SIM but not to telaprevir, boceprevir, or paritaprevir.[3] SIM RAVs in genotype 1a include R155K, R155K plus V36M, R155K plus Q80L, R155K plus S122R, R155K plus D168E, and preexisting Q80K. SIM RAVs in genotype 1b include D168V and Q80R plus D168E.[22]

The key RAVs in NS5A are located at position 28, 30, 31, and 93 (**Table 4**). The NS5A inhibitor in late-stage developments, daclatasvir, has resistant variants at L31V/M and Y93H/N.[28] Daclatasvir also has a resistant-associated polymorphism, Q30R/H. The NS5A inhibitor, LDV, when tested as monotherapy, has resistant variants: M28T, Q30R/H, L31 M, and Y93H/C in genotype 1a and only Y93H resistant variant in genotype 1b.[29,30] Preliminary data pooled from phase 2/3 trials of LDV/SOF suggest that the relapse rate is higher in individuals with baseline NS5A RAVs compared with those with no RAVs.[31] More information regarding the importance of testing for baseline RAVs with this regimen is still needed.

In the nucleoside inhibitor category, the drug SOF has a higher barrier to resistance compared with other categories of DAAs. The S282T resistant variant has shown in vitro resistance, which reduces viral fitness; but clinical resistance has not been clearly demonstrated in clinical trials.[22] Other NS5B substitutions, such as L159F and V321A, have been detected in patients who failed SOF-based clinical trials.[32] The high-resistance-barrier phenomenon of SOF seems useful in combination with other DAAs to compensate for resistance patterns of other drugs to achieve higher SVR rates.

Currently, an FDA-approved test is available to assess RAVs in the NS3/4a and NS5A coding region. Future tests assessing NS5A polymorphisms are likely to be available soon. Baseline testing may guide therapy in some situations or be used to explain relapse after therapy. Currently, the AASLD does not recommend baseline resistance testing. This concept is quickly evolving, however; based on observations in current treatment regimens, this may become a necessary part of regimen selection.

Viral factors, such as baseline viral load, have been implicated in the virologic nonresponse. Post hoc analysis of data from a phase 3 trial of SOF/LDV revealed a comparable high rate of SVR12 in treatment-naïve, noncirrhotic patients who were treated with 8 weeks of therapy compared with 12 weeks if the baseline HCV RNA viral load was less than 6,000,000 IU/mL.[33]

Host Factors

Host cytokines and the innate immune response play an important role in regulating HCV. Studies have shown various responses to HCV, with some individuals spontaneously clearing the virus on their own. Genetic polymorphisms, such as IL28B, regulate cytokine production, which may be associated with the variation in response to the virus. The role of polymorphism in tumor necrosis factor-α, transforming growth factor β-1, and IL-10 has been identified in chronic hepatitis C.[34] Single nucleotide polymorphism (SNPs) in a linkage disequilibrium block encompassing the 2 IFN-κ gene on chromosome 19 have been strongly linked to the response of PEG-IFN and RBV in many genotypes of hepatitis C.[34] From genome-wide associated studies, SNPs near the IL28B locus have also shown association with treatment response in patients with genotype 1 hepatitis C.[35] Slightly higher SVR rates have been seen in patients with the

Table 4
Resistance-associated variants in NS5A

	Genotype 1a								Genotype 1b					
	M28T	Q30R	Q30E	Q30H	L31M	Y93C	Y93H	Y93N	L28T	L31M	L31V/F	Q54H/N	Y93H	Y93N
Ombitasvir	+	+	−	−	−	+	+	+	−	−	+	−	+	−
LDV	+	+	+	+	+	+	+	+	+	+	+	−	+	+
Daclatasvir	+	+	+	+	+	+	+	+	+	+	+	+	+	+

There is significant overlap in the resistance of DAAs targeting NS5A for genotype 1a and 1b.
Data from Refs.[25–27]

favorable IL28B genotype CC compared with those with TT in IFN-free DAA trials[5]; however, appropriately powered studies designed to assess this are still lacking.

Other host factors that contribute to the antiviral nonresponse include age, sex, race, alcohol use, obesity, insulin resistance, hepatic steatosis, and vitamin D and vitamin B12 deficiencies.[36] Presence of hepatic steatosis has been shown in 547 patients treated with telaprevir/PEG/RBV to have lower SVR rates in patients with genotype 1.[36] Vitamin D status was previously shown to be associated with SVR rates; however, it is not known whether vitamin D or other predictors of IFN response will consistently impact IFN-free therapy.[37]

Altered Pharmacokinetics

Hepatic metabolism is key to multiple DAA drugs. If there is decreased hepatic metabolism in cases with extensive fibrosis or cirrhosis, it can disturb drug metabolism and lead to toxicity. RBV is metabolized in 2 pathways with reversible phosphorylation to monophosphate, diphosphate, and triphosphate metabolites in the nucleated cells and degradation involving deribosylation and amide hydrolysis to a triazole carboxamide.[38] There is no cytochrome P enzyme metabolism associated with RBV.

Reduced metabolism from drug-drug interactions or from poor hepatic or renal function may impact intracellular concentrations of the active drug. These were especially prominent in first-generation PIs.[39] SIM is metabolized by the CYP3A4 enzyme similar to telaprevir but to a lesser extent than boceprevir.[39] In contrast to the above-mentioned drugs, SOF has no metabolism from the CYP enzyme. It predominantly circulates in the inactive metabolite form, GS-331007, which is metabolized into active triphosphate GS-461203 via hydrolysis, phosphoramidate cleavage, and phosphorylation in the kidney. The active metabolite is then dephosphorylated to form GS-331007.[38] Because of the lack of metabolism via the CYP enzyme, SOF has no induction or inhibition of CYP enzymes and, thus, has no drug-drug interactions related to the CYP pathway. However, SOF is a substrate of transporter protein P-glycoprotein (pgP) and breast cancer resistance protein. Drugs that induce these pathways would decrease SOF therapeutic efficacy. Similar to SOF, LDV marginally affects the CYP enzyme. LDV is also a substrate of pgP; thus, drugs that induce the transporter protein pathway should also be avoided.[40] The key to achieving adequate serum levels of LDV and GS-5816 is an acid-rich environment in the gut.[40] Hence, proton pump inhibitor use may pose a problem.

Portosystemic Shunting and Cirrhosis

The liver plays a central role in the absorption, distribution, metabolism, and excretion of drugs and the drug pharmacokinetics, which can be influenced by the presence of cirrhosis. The mechanism of resistance in patients with advance liver fibrosis is not very clear. Decreased hepatic metabolism and portosystemic shunting has been associated with changes in the pharmacokinetics of drugs.

One study reported that malnutrition status of patients with advanced hepatitis C is associated with IFN resistance. They also showed that malnutrition impaired IFN signaling by inhibiting mammalian target of rapamycin complex 1 and activating the suppressor of cytokine signaling 3–mediated IFN inhibitory signaling through the nutrionsensing transcriptional factor forkhead box protein O3a.[41]

The mean area under the curve (AUC) of RBC is fairly similar in patients with Child-Pugh class A, B, and C cirrhosis as compared with controls.[38] However, the mean maximum peak plasma drug concentration level values increased with the severity of hepatic dysfunction and were 2 times greater in patients with Child-Pugh class B and C cirrhosis. This finding is evidenced by the close monitoring for side effects, such as anemia, which is recommended with RBV. Altered serum levels of DAAs in patients with reduced hepatic metabolism have also been seen. A study showed that after 7 days of exposure of SOF, the AUC was 126% and 143% higher in Child-Pugh class B and C, respectively, as compared with patients with normal hepatic function.[38] This finding suggests that, with advancing degrees of portal hypertension, response rates may decline.

THERAPEUTIC OPTIONS FOR RETREATMENT OF DIRECT-ACTING ANTIVIRAL FAILURES

Currently, 3 highly effective all oral, IFN-free DAA regimens are available for hepatitis C genotype 1. Limited data are available regarding retreatment in patients who are PI experienced, with either telaprevir or boceprevir. There is concern that resistance-associated variants in the NS3/4a region may be present in patients who were treated with a PI; thus, even second- and next-generation PIs are not indicated for patients who are PI experienced. A commercially available test assesses PI resistance, and this could inform the clinician whether baseline RAVs are present. Increasing data have become available for retreatment of patients who had been treated with SOF. A summary of regimens used for DAA failures is shown in **Fig. 2**.

Clinical Trials Inclusive of Sofosbuvir Failures in Genotype 1

The use of SOF with PEG-IFN/RBV for 12 weeks for genotype 1 or RBV alone for 24 weeks was the first FDA indication for this drug. Because of the high barrier to resistance and potency, retreatment with SOF seems to be much safer than with other DAAs. Initial evidence of this was published in a small cohort of patients with genotype 1 who failed 24 weeks of SOF plus RBV in the NIAID (National Institute of Allergy and Infectious Disease) SPARE study and were offered retreatment with 12 weeks of SOF/LDV in a small nonrandomized study.[42] Fourteen individuals participated, and most were African American (n = 13) and male (n = 13). The baseline characteristics of the group included 50% with advanced fibrosis (F3 and F4), and most (57%) were genotype 1a. A single patient was found to have the presence of the S282T polymorphism, which is the mutation that confers SOF resistance in vitro[46]; most patients had either CT or TT IL28B genotype status (86%). All attained undetectable HCV RNA by week 4 of therapy (rapid virologic response [RVR]), and all achieved SVR12 after completion of therapy.

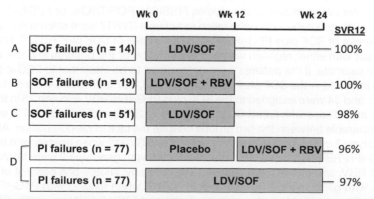

Fig. 2. Treatment regimens for genotype 1 DAA failures studied to date. Treatment duration and agents used is indicated in the rectangle, and SVR12 is shown on far right. (*Data from* Refs.[42–45])

In a partially randomized, open-label phase 2 study known as ELECTRON-2,[43] a subgroup of 19 patients who had received SOF prior were treated with 12 weeks of SOF/LDV plus RBV. The group was composed of noncirrhotic patients, including 17 of 19 individuals infected with genotype 1a. All patients treated with this regimen attained an RVR with no viral breakthrough on therapy, and 100% SVR12 was reported.

Recently, Wyles and colleagues[44] reported 51 SOF-experienced patients treated with PEG-IFN/RBV plus SOF, SOF/RBV, or SOF/placebo.[44] The cohort included some well-compensated cirrhotic patients (29%) and mostly genotype (GT) 1a patients (59%). Baseline resistance assay was performed, and no one demonstrated the SOF-associated RAV S282T. Although no patients were previously treated with a regimen containing an NS5A inhibitor, 12% were found to have baseline NS5A RAVs. Participants were treated with once-daily combination therapy SOF/LDV for 12 weeks. Ninety-eight percent were undetectable by week 4, and none experienced viral breakthrough on therapy. SVR was attained in 50 of 51 patients (98%). The single individual who relapsed was discovered to have been incorrectly genotyped and found to be infected with genotype 3a. This individual had been treated with SOF/RBV for 24 weeks before being retreated.

Perhaps one of the most complex groups of patients requiring retreatment is the PI-experienced cirrhotic group. Such a cohort of cirrhotic patients from France formerly enrolled in the CUPIC study[47] who failed both PEG-IFN/RBV and then later PEG-IFN/RBV plus PI (telaprevir or boceprevir) was treated with either 12 weeks of placebo followed by 12 weeks of SOF/LDV plus RBV (n = 77) or 24 weeks of SOF/LDV (n = 78).[45] No data were collected on baseline resistance; however, because the patients were not exposed to SOF or LDV, this was not anticipated to be a major factor. The two cohorts were well matched and had similar proportions of genotype 1a (62% vs 64%) and degree of hepatic function. Those treated with SOF/LDV plus RBV for 12 weeks had similar SVR12 rates as those treated with SOF/LDV for 24 weeks (96% vs 97%), and all showed modest improvement in liver function (albumin, bilirubin, and international normalized ratio). Individuals treated with SOF/LDV plus RBV had a 12-week lead-in of placebo, and the rates of adverse events in this group were similar to those treated with SOF/LDV plus RBV and 24 weeks of SOF/LDV. A single patient discontinued the study because of adverse events while on placebo; otherwise, treatment was generally well tolerated in all groups.

Retreatment of Sofosbuvir Failures with Genotype 2 or 3

Individuals who were treated in the studies FISSION, POSITRON, or FUSION (12 and 16 weeks) with genotype 2 or 3 who failed to achieve SVR12 were offered retreatment with 12 weeks of SOF plus PEG-IFN/RBV or 24 weeks of SOF plus RBV.[48] The decision to treat with either regimen was at the discretion of the patients and the investigator. For example, if the patients were determined to be intolerant to PEG-IFN, they could be included in the SOF plus RBV arm. Overall, 107 individuals were included in the study, and 34 were assigned to the SOF plus PEG-IFN/RBV arm and 73 in the SOF plus RBV arm. Those with IL28B CC status (32% vs 37%) and cirrhosis (41% vs 34%) were comparable between the two groups despite the lack of randomization. All those with genotype 2 infection (n = 4) achieved RVR and SVR12 when treated with the SOF plus PEG-IFN/RBV regimen. Two patients infected with genotype 2 were treated with SOF plus RBV, and one of them relapsed after therapy. Ninety-one percent of the individuals with genotype 3 (n = 22) attained SVR12 when treated with PEG-IFN/RBV plus SOF. Fewer patients with genotype 3 attained SVR12 (63%; n = 38). Cirrhosis seemed to be a major predictor of relapse in patients with genotype 3 treated with SOF plus RBV (SVR12: 74% vs 47%).

Approach to Patients Requiring Retreatment

Currently, there is no FDA-approved regimen for prior all-oral DAA treatment failures. Based on available data, SOF seems to be the cornerstone of salvage therapy, even when patients previously failed SOF. In patients with genotype 1, SOF may be combined with PEG-IFN/RBV, RBV alone, LDV, or LDV and RBV. The treatment duration has varied from 8 to 24 weeks. Currently, the only option for genotype 2 or 3 failures is longer duration of SOF and RBV or the addition of PEG-IFN to the regimen. Should daclatasvir obtain FDA approval, then it may improve the chance for SVR12, although this has not been studied.

There are no data to guide retreatment of the prior PI failure with second-generation PIs. Resistance testing for NS3/4A is available and can inform the clinician as to whether patients already have baseline resistance associated with intended PI of use; however, this has not been studied for efficacy. NS5A resistance testing is now available and could be of increasing utility as more patients fail future therapies using that class of drug. In vitro SOF resistance polymorphisms are known, such as S282T; this has recently been described also, although the significance is not yet clear.[49]

Should retreatment be considered, a conversation with patients should include the off-label use of the agents and make mention of the risk of acquisition of further resistance or retreatment failure. Fibrosis staging and knowledge of treatment history are important to determining therapy. Careful review of drug-drug interactions should be undertaken, and those concomitant medications that may diminish antiviral plasma levels should be avoided. Assessment of RAVs is relevant if patients are being retreated with a PI or NS5A inhibitor. Additionally, because third-party payers or outside pharmacies are involved, patients may have a delay on their 30-day refills. Therefore, anticipation of these complications is required. If noncompliance was suspected to have impacted prior DAA treatment, then strategies to improve this may impact subsequent treatment attempts. A strong patient-physician relationship and in-depth understanding of patients' psychosocial situations may reveal the causes for noncompliance.

Cocktail Mixology for Hepatitis C Virus

As resistance testing becomes more available, the rationale for combining agents from different manufacturers may gain importance. Some DAAs, such as SOF and SIM, can be prescribed individually; but others may be more difficult to combine because of packaging. The idea of creating individualized cocktails currently will be difficult on this basis; but as more agents become available, it may be a possibility. The combination of SOF, SIM, and daclatasvir is an example of such a cocktail that could be available shortly. Based on some promising clinical data, grazoprevir and elbasvir may also be combined with SOF in a similar fashion.[50] Combined use of LDV and SIM is not recommended because of potential drug-drug interactions. All of these potential combinations may need to be explored as new resistance patterns emerge, requiring combinations that may offer broader salvage options.

SUMMARY

HCV therapy has entered a new era. DAAs have revolutionized hepatitis C by increasing SVR rates from 50% to about 95% with improved patient tolerability and fewer adverse events. However, both patients and clinicians must demonstrate responsible use of these agents. The choice of drug combination should be impacted by multiple factors, such as patient selection, adverse-event profile of drugs, cost-effectiveness, comorbidities, and age of the patients. If patients fail, careful review of each case is required. The key to guiding clinicians in the future will be DAAs with FDA approval for salvage therapy and expansion of resistance testing.

REFERENCES

1. Scheel TK, Rice CM. Understanding the hepatitis C virus life cycle paves the way for highly effective therapies. Nat Med 2013;19:837–49.
2. Alter MJ. Epidemiology of hepatitis C. Hepatology (Baltimore, Md.) 1997;26: 62S–5S.
3. Manzano-Robleda Mdel C, Ornelas-Arroyo V, Barrientos-Gutierrez T, et al. Boceprevir and telaprevir for chronic genotype 1 hepatitis C virus infection. A systematic review and meta-analysis. Ann Hepatol 2015;14:46–57.
4. Beste LA, Green PK, Ioannou GN. Boceprevir and telaprevir-based regimens for the treatment of hepatitis C virus in HIV/HCV coinfected patients. Eur J Gastroenterol Hepatol 2015;27:123–9.
5. Lawitz E, Sulkowski MS, Ghalib R, et al. Simeprevir plus sofosbuvir, with or without ribavirin, to treat chronic infection with hepatitis C virus genotype 1 in nonresponders to pegylated interferon and ribavirin and treatment-naive patients: the COSMOS randomised study. Lancet 2014;384:1756–65.
6. Poordad F, McCone J Jr, Bacon BR, et al. Boceprevir for untreated chronic HCV genotype 1 infection. New Engl J Med 2011;364:1195–206.
7. Bacon BR, Gordon SC, Lawitz E, et al. Boceprevir for previously treated chronic HCV genotype 1 infection. New Engl J Med 2011;364:1207–17.
8. Jacobson IM, McHutchison JG, Dusheiko G, et al. Telaprevir for previously untreated chronic hepatitis C virus infection. New Engl J Med 2011;364: 2405–16.
9. Zeuzem S, Andreone P, Pol S, et al. Telaprevir for retreatment of HCV infection. New Engl J Med 2011;364:2417–28.
10. Manns MP, Markova AA, Calle Serrano B, et al. Phase III results of boceprevir in treatment naive patients with chronic hepatitis C genotype 1. Liver Int 2012; 32(Suppl 1):27–31.
11. Price JC, Murphy RC, Shvachko VA, et al. Effectiveness of telaprevir and boceprevir triple therapy for patients with hepatitis C virus infection in a large integrated care setting. Dig Dis Sci 2014;59:3043–52.
12. Ioannou GN, Beste LA, Green PK. Similar effectiveness of boceprevir and telaprevir treatment regimens for hepatitis C virus infection on the basis of a nationwide study of veterans. Clin Gastroenterol Hepatol 2014;12:1371–80.
13. Hezode C, Fontaine H, Dorival C, et al. Effectiveness of telaprevir or boceprevir in treatment-experienced patients with HCV genotype 1 infection and cirrhosis. Gastroenterology 2014;147(1):132–42.e4.
14. Bonnet D, Guivarch M, Berard E, et al. Telaprevir- and boceprevir-based tritherapies in real practice for F3-F4 pretreated hepatitis C virus patients. World J Hepatol 2014;6:660–9.
15. Jacobson IM, Dore GJ, Foster GR, et al. Simeprevir with pegylated interferon alfa 2a plus ribavirin in treatment-naive patients with chronic hepatitis C virus genotype 1 infection (QUEST-1): a phase 3, randomised, double-blind, placebo-controlled trial. Lancet 2014;384:403–13.
16. Manns M, Marcellin P, Poordad F, et al. Simeprevir with pegylated interferon alfa 2a or 2b plus ribavirin in treatment-naive patients with chronic hepatitis C virus genotype 1 infection (QUEST-2): a randomised, double-blind, placebo-controlled phase 3 trial. Lancet 2014;384:414–26.

17. Lawitz E, Mangia A, Wyles D, et al. Sofosbuvir for previously untreated chronic hepatitis C infection. New Engl J Med 2013;368:1878–87.
18. Jensen D, Pockros P, Sherman K, et al. Safety and efficacy of sofosbuvir-containing regimens for hepatitis c: real-world experience in a diverse, longitudinal observational cohort. Hepatology 2014;60(Suppl 1):219A–20A [abstract: 45].
19. Dieterich D, Flamm S, Kowdley K, et al. Evaluation of sofosbuvir and simeprevir-based regimens in the TRIO network: academic and community treatment of a real-world, heterogeneous population. Hepatology 2014;60(Suppl 1):220A [abstract: 46].
20. Ji H, Kozak RA, Biondi MJ, et al. Next generation sequencing of the hepatitis C virus NS5B gene reveals potential novel S282 drug resistance mutations. Virology 2015;477C:1–9.
21. Fishman SL, Branch AD. The quasispecies nature and biological implications of the hepatitis C virus. Infect Genet Evol 2009;9(6):1158–67.
22. Wyles DL, Gutierrez JA. Importance of HCV genotype 1 subtypes for drug resistance and response to therapy. J viral Hepat 2014;21:229–40.
23. Pilot-Matias T, Tripathi R, Cohen D, et al. In vitro and in vivo antiviral activity and resistance profile of the hepatitis C virus NS3/4A protease inhibitor ABT-450. Antimicrob Agents Chemother 2015;59:988–97.
24. Summa V, Ludmerer SW, McCauley JA, et al. MK-5172, a selective inhibitor of hepatitis C virus NS3/4a protease with broad activity across genotypes and resistant variants. Antimicrob Agents Chemother 2012;56:4161–7.
25. Plaza Z, Soriano V, Vispo E, et al. Prevalence of natural polymorphisms at the HCV NS5A gene associated with resistance to daclatasvir, an NS5A inhibitor. Antivir Ther 2012;17:921–6.
26. Nakamoto S, Kanda T, Wu S, et al. Hepatitis C virus NS5A inhibitors and drug resistance mutations. World J Gastroenterol 2014;20:2902–12.
27. Krishnan P, Beyer J, Mistry N, et al. In vitro and in vivo antiviral activity and resistance profile of ombitasvir, an inhibitor of hepatitis C virus NS5A. Antimicrob Agents Chemother 2015;59:979–87.
28. McPhee F, Hernandez D, Yu F, et al. Resistance analysis of hepatitis C virus genotype 1 prior treatment null responders receiving daclatasvir and asunaprevir. Hepatology (Baltimore, Md.) 2013;58:902–11.
29. Wong KA, Worth A, Martin R, et al. Characterization of hepatitis C virus resistance from a multiple-dose clinical trial of the novel NS5A inhibitor GS-5885. Antimicrob Agents Chemother 2013;57:6333–40.
30. Dvory-Sobol H, Doehle B, Svarovskaia E, et al. The prevalence of HCV NS5A, nucleoside and protease inhibitor resistance associated variants and the effects on treatment with ledipasvir/sofosbuvir ± RBV in the phase 3 ION studies. International Workshop on Antiviral Drug Resistance. 2014. [abstract# 10]; P3.
31. Sarrazin C, Dvory-Sobol H, Svarovskaia E, et al. The prevalence and the effect of HCV NS5A resistance-associated variants in patients with compensated cirrhosis treated with ledipasvir/sofosbuvir ± RBV. J Hepatol 2015;62:S622.
32. Donaldson EF, Harrington PR, O'Rear JJ, et al. Clinical evidence and bioinformatics characterization of potential hepatitis C virus resistance pathways for sofosbuvir. Hepatology (Baltimore, Md.) 2015;61:56–65.
33. Kowdley KV, Gordon SC, Reddy KR, et al. Ledipasvir and sofosbuvir for 8 or 12 weeks for chronic HCV without cirrhosis. New Engl J Med 2014;370:1879–88.
34. Pasha HF, Radwan MI, Hagrass HA, et al. Cytokines genes polymorphisms in chronic hepatitis C: impact on susceptibility to infection and response to therapy. Cytokines 2013;61:478–84.

35. Ge D, Fellay J, Thompson AJ, et al. Genetic variation in IL28B predicts hepatitis C treatment-induced viral clearance. Nature 2009;461:399–401.

36. Zhu Y, Chen S. Antiviral treatment of hepatitis C virus infection and factors affecting efficacy. World J Gastroenterol 2013;19:8963–73.

37. Gutierrez JA, Parikh N, Branch AD. Classical and emerging roles of vitamin d in hepatitis C virus infection. Semin Liver Dis 2011;31:387–98.

38. de Kanter CT, Drenth JP, Arends JE, et al. Viral hepatitis C therapy: pharmacokinetic and pharmacodynamic considerations. Clin Pharmacokinet 2014;53: 409–27.

39. Kiser JJ, Burton JR Jr, Everson GT. Drug-drug interactions during antiviral therapy for chronic hepatitis C. Nature reviews. Gastroenterol Hepatol 2013;10: 596–606.

40. Soriano V, Labarga P, Barreiro P, et al. Drug interactions with new hepatitis C oral drugs. Expert Opin Drug Metab Toxicol 2015;11:333–41.

41. Shirasaki T, Honda M, Shimakami T, et al. Impaired interferon signaling in chronic hepatitis C patients with advanced fibrosis via the transforming growth factor beta signaling pathway. Hepatology (Baltimore, Md.) 2014;60:1519–30.

42. Osinusi A, Kohli A, Marti MM, et al. Re-treatment of chronic hepatitis C virus genotype 1 infection after relapse: an open-label pilot study. Ann Intern Med 2014; 161:634–8.

43. Gane E, Hyland R, An D, et al. Sofosbuvir/ledipasvir fixed dose combination is safe and effective in difficult-to-treat populations including genotype-3 patients, decompensated genotype-1 patients, and genotype-1 patients with prior sofosbuvir treatment experience. J Hepatol 2014: S1–3. 49th Annual Meeting of the European Association for the Study of the Liver: Abstract 06.

44. Wyles D, Pockros P, Zhu Y, et al. Retreatment of patients who failed prior sofosbuvir-based regimens with all oral fixed-dose combination ledipasvir/sofosbuvir plus ribavirin for 12 weeks. Hepatology 2014: A235. 65th Annual Meeting of the American Association for the Study of Liver Diseases.

45. Bourliere M, Bronowicki J, de Ledinghen V, et al. Ledipasvir/sofosbuvir fixed dose combination is safe and efficacious in cirrhotic patients who have previously failed protease-inhibitor based triple therapy. Hepatology 2014. 65th Annual Meeting of the American Association for the Study of Liver Diseases:LB-6.

46. Lam AM, Espiritu C, Bansal S, et al. Genotype and subtype profiling of PSI-7977 as a nucleotide inhibitor of hepatitis C virus. Antimicrob Agents Chemother 2012; 56:3359–68.

47. Hezode C, Fontaine H, Dorival C, et al. Triple therapy in treatment-experienced patients with HCV-cirrhosis in a multicentre cohort of the French Early Access Programme (ANRS CO20-CUPIC) - NCT01514890. J Hepatol 2013;59:434–41.

48. Esteban B, Nyberg L, Lalezari J, et al. Successful retreatment with sofosbuvir-containing regimens for HCV genotype 2 or 3 infected patients who failed prior sofosbuvir plus ribavirin therapy. J Hepatol 2014. European Association for the Study of the Liver: S4–S5.

49. Lawitz E, Flamm S, Yang J, et al. Retreatment of patients who failed 8 or 12 weeks of ledipasvir/sofosbuvir-based regimens with ledipasvir/sofosbuvir for 24 weeks. J Hepatol 2015. EASL - The International Liver Congress 2015:O005.

50. Lawitz E, Poordad F, Gutierrez J, et al. C-SWIFT: grazoprevir (MK-5172) + elbasvir (MK-8742) + sofosbuvir in treatment-naive patients with hepatitis C virus genotype 1 infection, with and without cirrhosis, for durations of 4, 6, or 8 weeks (interim results). Hepatology 2014. 65th Annual Meeting of the American Association for the Study of Liver Diseases: LB-33.

Regimens for Cirrhotic Patients

Paul Y. Kwo, MD

KEYWORDS

- Direct-acting antivirals • Hepatitis C • Cirrhosis • Sofosbuvir • Ledipasvir
- Paritaprevir • Ombitasvir • Simeprevir

KEY POINTS

- It is now expected that patients with compensated cirrhosis will achieve sustained virologic response (SVR) rates similar to those who do not have cirrhosis.
- The most significant population requiring new therapies is the genotype 3 treatment-experienced cirrhotic patients, in whom the optimal therapy remains unclear.
- Once SVR is achieved, patients should continue to be monitored for complications, including varices, decompensation, and hepatocellular carcinoma.

Hepatitis C is a blood-borne virus that is found worldwide. Although precise epidemiologic data are not available it is estimated that there are 150 million persons globally who have chronic hepatitis C infection and 350,000 to 500,000 people die each year from hepatitis C–related liver diseases.[1] In the United States, the prevalence is 1.8% and recent estimates suggest that as many as 5 million individuals may be infected with chronic hepatitis C.[2] By the year 2020, it is estimated that there may be 1 million individuals with hepatitis C who have progressed to cirrhosis.[3] Hepatitis C infection progressing to cirrhosis is the most common cause of hepatocellular carcinoma in United States and the most common indication for orthotopic liver transplant worldwide. A recent estimate has suggested that effective therapy for hepatitis C could potentially substantially reduce the transplant requirement for those with chronic hepatitis C.[4]

In the evaluation of chronic hepatitis C, it is essential to assess for the presence or absence of cirrhosis. Historically, this has been achieved with liver biopsy, which is considered the goal standard. Recently, elastography has been approved in the United States, which allows a noninvasive measure of cirrhosis (for hepatitis C >12.5 kPa).[5] Moreover, serum markers of fibrosis are also available. In addition, imaging may also be used to show cirrhosis and, with a nodular liver, cirrhotic

Dr P.Y. Kwo has received grant support and served on advisory boards for Abbvie, BMS, Gilead, Merck, and Janssen.
Gastroenterology/Hepatology Division, Liver Transplantation, Indiana University Health, Indiana University School of Medicine, 975 West Walnut, IB 327, Indianapolis, IN 46202-5121, USA
E-mail address: pkwo@iu.edu

morphology and portal hypertension, all pointing to a diagnosis of cirrhosis. Once cirrhosis is diagnosed, these patients should be screened regularly for hepatocellular carcinoma with ultrasonography every 6 months.[6] Endoscopy should also be performed to assess for the absence or presence of varices.[7] The recent American Association for the Study of Liver Diseases (AASLD)/Infectious Diseases Society of America (IDSA) guideline (http://www.hcvguidelines.org/) confirms the importance of assessing for cirrhosis.

The treatment of chronic hepatitis C infection has undergone a revolution in the past 2 years. In December 2013, the first oral regimen, sofosbuvir and ribavirin, was approved without interferon for genotypes 2 and 3 based on 3 registration studies.[8–10] Moreover, the combination of 2 medicines, sofosbuvir and simeprevir, which were approved separately for the treatment of hepatitis C genotype 1 in 2013, could be combined with or without ribavirin for a genotype 1 all-oral regimen to be given with high sustained response rates.[11] Historically, lower sustained response rates have been observed in cirrhotic patients who received peginterferon with or without direct-acting antiviral agents (DAAs).[12–14] As treatment have evolved to all-oral regimens, many of the previous predictors of poor treatment response, such as race, viral level, and IL28B genotype, that predicted poor response to peginterferon and ribavirin no longer predict poor response to all-oral therapies with direct-acting antiviral agents for hepatitis C. However, even in this current era, patients with cirrhosis and advanced liver disease remain a population that may require additional strategies to achieve sustained virologic response (SVR) compared with those without cirrhosis. This requirement is particularly important because sustained response in this population has significant clinical impact with the potential to help fibrosis progression, reduce the risk of decompensation and liver cancer, and possibly prevent progression of chronic liver disease to a point at which orthotopic liver transplant must be considered.[15] However, in patients with Child A cirrhosis, the population that is discussed here, no dose adjustments are required for any of the DAA classes or ribavirin. Therapy in patients with Child B/C cirrhosis is discussed elsewhere in this issue.

TREATMENT OPTIONS: GENOTYPE 1

The treatment options for patients with hepatitis C differ by genotype. Historically, genotype 1 has been most the difficult genotype to treat. There are currently 3 approved treatment options for genotype 1 and all 3 treatment options may be used in patients with hepatitis C with cirrhosis in the United States. The treatment options for treatment-naive patients with cirrhosis are listed in **Table 1** and include sofosbuvir and ledipasvir for 12 weeks, sofosbuvir plus simeprevir for 24 weeks, and paritaprevir plus ombitasvir plus dasabuvir with ribavirin for 12 to 24 weeks depending on genotype 1 subtype (1a or 1b). The data for these recommendations come from landmark

| Table 1 | | | |
| Genotype 1 regimens for patients with compensated cirrhosis | | | |
Treatment Naive	1a/1b	Duration (wk)	SVR (n/N)
Sofosbuvir + ledipasvir	1a/1b	12	94% (32 of 34)
Paritaprevir/r + ombitasvir + dasabuvir + RBV	1a	24	93% (52 of 56)
Paritaprevir/r + ombitasvir + dasabuvir + RBV	1b	12	100% (22 of 22)
Sofosbuvir + simeprevir ± RBV	1a/1b	24	100% (3 of 3) + RBV 100% (5 of 5) no RBV

Abbreviation: RBV, ribavirin.

studies that evaluated the combinations of DAAs for the treatment of hepatitis C. The ION-1 study evaluated sofosbuvir/ledipasvir as a fixed-dose combination with and without ribavirin for 12-week and 24-week durations.[16] In the cirrhotic cohorts, 12 weeks of ledipasvir or sofosbuvir led to an SVR rate of 94% (32 of 34), with the 24-week duration arm achieving an SVR of 97% (31 of 32). The treatment failures were all related to relapse or being lost to follow-up.

The TURQUOISE-II study evaluated paritaprevir, ombitasvir, dasabuvir in combination with weight-based ribavirin for 12 or 24 weeks in patients with cirrhosis.[17] The treatment-naive SVR rates in genotype 1a were 92% and 93% for 12 and 24 weeks respectively versus 100% in those with genotype 1b regardless of treatment duration. Treatment failure in the genotype 1a cohort was primarily caused by relapse occurring in the 12-week arms in 12 of 203 individuals versus 1 of 164 individuals who received the 24-week duration of therapy. Breakthrough was rare, with just 1 individual in the 12-week arm having breakthrough and 3 in the 24-week arm having breakthrough. The resistant associated variants observed included D168V (NS3) and Q30R (NS5A) and were seen most frequently in patients infected with GT1a.

In addition, the combination of sofosbuvir and simeprevir has been approved based on the recently published phase II COSMOS study.[11] In this study, a total of 8 individuals who were cirrhotic and treatment naive were enrolled with SVR rates of 100% in those who received sofosbuvir and simeprevir or sofosbuvir or simeprevir with ribavirin for a 24-week duration. Phase III trials are fully enrolled and results are expected in 2015. Based on the small amount of data for treatment-naive individuals with cirrhosis, the 24-week treatment course with sofosbuvir and simeprevir is recommended.

Treatment Options for Genotype 1 Individuals Who Have Failed Previous Therapy

For patients who have failed therapy with peginterferon, and ribavirin with or without DAAs, there are multiple excellent options for those with compensated cirrhosis. The current guidelines recommended for those with compensated cirrhosis who failed therapy with peginterferon and ribavirin include ledipasvir or sofosbuvir for genotypes 1a and 1b, 24 weeks; or ledipasvir or sofosbuvir plus weight-based ribavirin for 12 weeks; paritaprevir, ombitasvir, or dasabuvir with weight-based ribavirin for 24 weeks for genotype 1a infection and for 12 weeks for those with 1b cirrhosis; or sofosbuvir or simeprevir with or without ribavirin for 24 weeks for genotypes 1a and 1b. For those with cirrhosis who have failed peginterferon, ribavirin, and a first-generation protease inhibitor regimen (with telaprevir or boceprevir), ledipasvir and sofosbuvir for 24 weeks or ledipasvir and sofosbuvir plus ribavirin 1000 to 1200 mg for 12 weeks are recommended treatment options (**Table 2**). These recommendations come from 2 pivotal phase 3 studies and additional smaller studies. The ION-2 study evaluated the efficacy of sofosbuvir and ledipasvir and enrolled 444 patients in a similar design to the treatment-naive ION-1 study with a total of 88 patients with cirrhosis.[18] In patients in the cirrhotic cohorts who failed peginterferon and ribavirin, 12 weeks of sofosbuvir/ledipasvir led to an overall SVR rate of 88% (7 of 8) and 78% (7 of 9) without or with ribavirin, which was significantly lower than the 100% (17 of 17) SVR rates noted in the 24-week treatment arms with or without ribavirin. However, the cohort size was small in all of these arms. It was from this ION-2 study that the 24-week duration of therapy was recommended for treatment nonresponders with hepatitis C with sofosbuvir/ledipasvir.

For patients who failed peginterferon, ribavirin, and a protease inhibitor, the combination of sofosbuvir/ledipasvir for 24 weeks is the US Food and Drug Administration (FDA)–recommended treatment option, with sofosbuvir/ledipasvir for 24 weeks or sofosbuvir/ledipasvir with ribavirin 1000 to 1200 mg for 12 weeks being treatment

Table 2
Genotype 1 regimens for patients with compensated cirrhosis who have failed previous therapy

	1a/1b	Duration (wk)	SVR (n/N)
Treatment Failure PEG-IFN/RBV			
Sofosbuvir + ledipasvir	1a/1b	24	100% (8 of 8)
Sofosbuvir + ledipasvir + RBV	1a/1b	12	78% (7 of 9)
Paritaprevir/r + ombitasvir + dasabuvir + RBV[a]	1a	24	95% (59 of 62)
Paritaprevir/r + ombitasvir + dasabuvir + RBV	1b	12	98% (45 of 46)
Sofosbuvir + simeprevir ± RBV	1a/1b	24	100% (9 of 9) + RBV 100% (4 of 4) no RBV
Treatment Failure PEG-IFN/RBV + PI			
Sofosbuvir + ledipasvir	1a/1b	24	100% (14 of 14) 97% (75 of 77)
Sofosbuvir + ledipasvir + RBV	1a/1b	12	96% (74 of 77)
Treatment Failure PEG-IFN/RBV + SOF			
Sofosbuvir + ledipasvir + RBV	1a/1b	12	100% (15 of 15)

Abbreviations: PEG-IFN, peginterferon; PI, protease inhibitor.
[a] SVR of 93% for G1a null responders, 100% for other groups.

options recommended by the joint AASLD/IDSA guidelines. These data are derived in part from the ION-2 study in which a total of 54 cirrhotic patients who failed first-generation protease inhibitors were enrolled. The overall SVR rates for cirrhotic patients in the 12-week arms were 86% (12 of 14) and 85% (11 of 13) without and with ribavirin versus 100% (27 of 27) in the 24-week arms regardless of ribavirin use. These results led to the FDA approval for 24 weeks of sofosbuvir and ledipasvir for protease failures without ribavirin. A recent report of a large French cohort of patients who failed both peginterferon ribavirin and peginterferon and first-generation protease showed overall SVR rates of 97% for those who received ledipasvir/sofosbuvir for 24 weeks versus 96% for those who received ledipasvir/sofosbuvir and ribavirin 1000 to 1200 mg for 12 weeks.[19] Cirrhosis was determined by biopsy; FibroScan score greater than 12.5 kPa; FibroTest score greater 0.75; or an AST to platelet ratio index of greater than 2. Based on these findings, both 12-week treatment duration with ribavirin and 24 weeks without ribavirin are treatment options that are recommended by the joint AASLD/IDSA guidelines committee for cirrhotic patients who are candidates for therapy with sofosbuvir/ledipasvir. In addition, for genotype 1 patients who have failed sofosbuvir therapies, a preliminary report showed a high sustained response rate with 12 weeks of sofosbuvir/ledipasvir with ribavirin 1000 to 1200 mg daily for 12 weeks. In this study, 15 of 50 genotype 1 individuals with cirrhosis were retreated with sofosbuvir/ledipasvir with ribavirin, with all 15 achieving SVR.[20]

The combination of paritaprevir, ombitasvir, dasabuvir with ribavirin has also been studied in peginterferon and ribavirin failures without protease exposure. This analysis is derived from the previously mentioned TURQUOISE study, which assessed this combination for 12 and 24 weeks with ribavirin. For genotype 1a, high SVR rates were seen in all cirrhotic patients except genotype 1a null responders, and the SVR rate was 80% in the 12-week treatment arm. In the 24-week treatment arms, high SVR rates were see across all types of nonresponders: relapsers, 100% (13 of 13); partial responders, 100% (10 of 10); and null responders, 93% (39 of 42). High SVR rates were seen in the 12-week groups except for null responders: relapsers, 93% (14 of 15); partial responders, 100% (11 of 10); and null responders, 80% (40 of 40). For genotype 1b, uniformly high SVR rates were seen regardless of 12-week or 24-week duration, with just 1 partial nonresponder failing to achieve SVR in the 12-week or 24 week arms. Thus, for genotype 1a, to maximize SVR, 24 weeks of paritaprevir, ombitasvir, dasabuvir with ribavirin should be administered, although there are likely to be genotype 1a subgroups that will have their therapy truncated at 12 weeks of therapy (more data are required). For genotype 1b, 12 weeks of treatment with paritaprevir, ombitasvir, dasabuvir, and ribavirin should lead to high rates without sacrificing SVR in all types of nonresponders. For genotype 1b cirrhosis patients, an important question that is being addressed is whether ribavirin is required; this study is ongoing (NCT02167945).

For the combination of sofosbuvir and simeprevir the data also come from the phase II COSMOS study and included a total of 22 patients who received simeprevir or sofosbuvir with or without ribavirin for 12 or 24 weeks. Again, 100% SVR rates were seen in the 24-week duration, although the population size is small (13) versus 8 of 9 individuals who received treatment for 12 weeks and who achieved SVR. Again, larger phase III trials are fully enrolled, but, based on these limited data, it was recommended that 24 weeks of sofosbuvir/simeprevir with or without ribavirin 1000 to 1200 mg should be administered.

GENOTYPE 2

The current standard of care for genotype 2 hepatitis C is sofosbuvir and ribavirin for 12 weeks. A 16-week duration is recommended for patients with genotype 2 in whom peginterferon and ribavirin have failed, with an alternative regimen being peginterferon and ribavirin with sofosbuvir for 12 weeks. In genotype 2 patients with cirrhosis, extension of treatment to 16 weeks is recommended in both treatment-naive and treatment-experienced patients with cirrhosis, although there are no prospective clinical trial data that have evaluated this approach (http://www.hcvguidelines.org/). The recommendation comes from an interim analysis from a payer network from real-world data that has shown higher SVR rates in treatment naive patients who receive 16 weeks of therapy versus 12 weeks, although the final analyses are not yet complete.[21] For genotype 2 treatment failures with cirrhosis, current AASLD/IDSA guidelines recommend that clinicians should treat for 16 weeks in patients who have failed therapy with peginterferon and ribavirin. Two studies have given conflicting results. The Phase 3 Fusion study noted that cirrhotic patients with genotype 2 who failed previous therapy had improved SVR rates with extension from 12 to 16 weeks of sofosbuvir/ribavirin (from 60% to 78%).[22] However, a subsequent German study showed that infected individuals with cirrhosis with genotype 2 could achieve an overall SVR rate of 88% with just 12 weeks of sofosbuvir and ribavirin.[9] It is this author's preference to offer cirrhotic naive and nonresponders 16 weeks of therapy. In addition, another option is 12 weeks of peginterferon, ribavirin, and sofosbuvir for 12 weeks based on a study that showed that triple therapy allowed genotype 2 nonresponders to achieve an SVR rate of 92.9% (13 of 14). Although the trend of therapy is toward removal of interferon from options, this remains another treatment choice for those patients with cirrhosis who can tolerate interferon.[9]

GENOTYPE 3

Genotype 3 has become the most problematic genotype in which to achieve SVR and this difficulty is particularly reflected in those with cirrhosis (**Table 3**). For genotype 3,

Table 3
Therapy options for genotype 3 patients with cirrhosis

Treatment Naive	Duration (wk)	SVR (n/N)
Sofosbuvir + ribavirin 1000–1200 mg	24	92% (12 of 13)
Sofosbuvir + daclatasvir	12	58% (11 of 19)
Treatment Failure PEG-IFN/RBV		
Sofosbuvir + daclatasvir	12	69% (9 of 13)
Sofosbuvir + ribavirin 1000–1200 mg	24	60% (27 of 45)
Sofosbuvir + PEG-IFN + RBV 1000–1200 mg	12	83% (10 of 12)
Sofosbuvir + ledipasvir + RBV 1000–1200 mg	12	73% (16 of 22)

the current recommended treatment is sofosbuvir 400 mg with weight-based ribavirin 1000 to 1200 mg for 24 weeks in those with and without cirrhosis. This 24-week duration is based on the Valence study, which included 250 treatment-naive and treatment-experienced subjects with genotype 3 infection in Germany.[9] The overall SVR rate was 84% with higher SVR rates seen in treatment-naive subjects than in treatment-experienced genotype 3 patients (93% vs 77%). For those with genotype 3 infection and cirrhosis, treatment-naive patients achieved an SVR rate of 92% (12 of 13) but treatment-experienced cirrhotic patients had a marked reduction in SVR rates to 60% (27 of 45). These SVR results were higher than the SVR rates reported with 12-week or 16-week regimens in the Fission and Fusion studies, in which SVR rates ranged from 63% in the treatment-naive genotype 3 population to 30% and 60% respectively in the treatment-experienced population with 12 and 16 weeks of sofosbuvir and ribavirin. Nonetheless, treatment-experienced genotype 3 patients with cirrhosis remain a problematic population. An alternative treatment regimen that is recommended with currently approved therapies includes triple therapy with the combination of peginterferon alfa with ribavirin and sofosbuvir for 12 weeks in patients who can tolerate retreatment with interferon based on a recent report in which genotype 3 cirrhotic patients who were retreated with peginterferon, ribavirin, and sofosbuvir achieved a sustained response rate of 83% (10 of 12).[9]

For genotype 3 cirrhotic patients, other treatment options have been explored. Single-center studies have examined the efficacy of ledipasvir, which has a markedly higher EC50 (concentration that gives half-maximal response) for genotype 3 (168 nM) than for genotypes 1a/1b (0.031 nM/0.004 nM), and sofosbuvir with ribavirin 1000 to 1200 mg for 12 weeks for cirrhotic genotype 3 individuals. In a recent report, 16 of 22 patients with genotype 3 cirrhosis who failed interferon-based therapy achieved SVR for an overall SVR of 73%.[2] Another strategy has been to combine the NS5a inhibitor daclatasvir with sofosbuvir without ribavirin for 12 weeks. Daclatasvir is approved in parts of Europe and Japan and has an EC50 for genotype 3a of less than or equal to 1.25 nM (http://www.ema.europa.eu/docs/en_GB/document_library/Other/2014/02/WC500160498.pdf). The phase 3 Ally study examined the efficacy of daclatasvir and sofosbuvir for 12 weeks without ribavirin. In this study, 19 of 101 treatment-naive individuals and 13 of 51 treatment-experienced individuals were cirrhotic.[4] The overall SVR rate in cirrhosis for 12 weeks of sofosbuvir and daclatasvir was 62% (20 of 32) with a treatment-naive SVR rate of 58% (11 of 19) and a treatment-experienced SVR rate of 69% (9 of 13). Two trials are planned to assess the efficacy of daclatasvir, sofosbuvir, and ribavirin for durations from 12 to 16 or 16 to 24 weeks in genotype 3 cirrhotic patients (NCT02319031 and NCT02304159). Preliminary data with sofosbuvir and the NS5a inhibitor GS5816 seem promising, with phase 3 trials underway in patients with cirrhosis. At present, treatment-naive cirrhotic individuals may be treated with sofosbuvir and ribavirin for 24 weeks with an expectation of a high SVR rates. However, treatment-experienced cirrhotic genotype 3 individuals remain a population in need of new strategies. SVR rates remain disappointing in treatment-experienced patients with cirrhosis. Longer durations of therapy for treatment with second-generation NS5A inhibitors in combination with other DAAs are likely to be required to achieve the same success as has been seen in genotypes 1 and 2.

GENOTYPE 4

Genotype 4 is commonly found in the Middle East and northern Africa. Historically, peginterferon and ribavirin for 36 to 48 weeks has been the treatment of choice, with sustained response rates that are higher than for genotype 1 but lower than for genotypes 2 and 3.[23] Compared with genotypes 1, 2, and 3, there are few data available in genotype 4, with fewer data available in those with cirrhosis. Three all-oral DAA combination therapies for genotype 4 are currently recommended, including paritaprevir, ombitasvir, and weight-based ribavirin for 12 weeks, ledipasvir and sofosbuvir for 12 weeks, or sofosbuvir and ribavirin for 24 weeks (**Table 4**).

The recommendation for paritaprevir, ombitasvir, and weight-based ribavirin is based on the phase 2B PEARL-1 study that included 86 treatment-naive individuals with or without cirrhosis who were randomized to receive paritaprevir and ombitasvir with or without ribavirin for 12 weeks, with 5 patients having F3 fibrosis or higher.[24] The SVR rate in the paritaprevir, ombitasvir, and ribavirin arm was 100% versus 91% without ribavirin. The PEARL-1 study also treated 49 genotype 4 nonresponders in a single arm with paritaprevir, ombitasvir, and ribavirin, with the SVR rate again being 100% with 5 patients with F3 fibrosis or higher. The combination of sofosbuvir/ledipasvir was evaluated in the SYNERGY trial, in which 21 genotype 4 infected individuals were treated for 12 weeks, 7 of the 21 having cirrhosis. The overall SVR rate was 95%, with 1 patient who failed having withdrawn consent (did not have cirrhosis), and the other 20 patients achieving SVR.[25] Sofosbuvir plus weight-based ribavirin for 24 weeks is another option for genotype 4 patients. A recent report randomized 60 genotype 4 patients who were either treatment naive or treatment experienced to receive 12 or

Table 4		
Treatment options for genotypes 4, 5, and 6		
Treatment of Genotype 4 Naive	Duration (wk)	SVR (n/N)
Paritaprevir/r + ombitasvir + RBV	12	100% (5 of 5)[a]
Sofosbuvir + ledipasvir	12	100% (4 of 4)
Sofosbuvir + ribavirin 1000–1200 mg	24	100% (3 of 3)
Genotype 4 Treatment Failure PEG-IFN/RBV		
Paritaprevir/r + ombitasvir + RBV	12	100% (5 of 5)[a]
Sofosbuvir + PEG-IFN + RBV	12	83% (10 of 12)
Sofosbuvir + ledipasvir	12	100% (3 of 3)
Genotype 5		
Sofosbuvir + PEG-IFN + RBV 1000–1200 mg	12	No data
Genotype 6		
Sofosbuvir + ledipasvir	12	100% (2 of 2)

[a] Patients had F3/F4 fibrosis.

Table 5
On-treatment monitoring: genotype 1 with cirrhosis

Treatment Week	1	2	4	8	12/EOT	16[a]	20[a]	24[a]	SVR 12
CBC	X[a]	X[a]	X	X	X	X	X	X	—
Creatinine	—	—	X	X	X	X	X	X	—
Calculated GFR	—	—	X	X	X	X	X	X	—
Hepatic fxn panel	—	—	X	X	X	X	X	X	—
TSH (with IFN)	—	—	—	—	X	—	—	X	—
HCV RNA	—	—	X	—	X	—	—	X	X

Safety data from phase II/III studies suggest that no difference in monitoring is required for patients with Child A cirrhosis.

Assessments for drug-related adverse effects should be conducted more frequently if clinically indicated in patients receiving RBV.

Abbreviations: CBC, complete blood count; EOT, end of treatment; fxn, function; GFR, glomerular filtration rate; HCV, hepatitis C virus; TSH, thyroid-stimulating hormone.

[a] Consider CBC at weeks 1 and 2 if using ribavirin with hemoglobin (Hgb) level less than 12 g/dL or GFR less than 60 mL/min.

24 weeks of sofosbuvir plus weight-based ribavirin.[26] High SVR rates of 93% were seen in the 24-week treatment arm (27 of 29), with all 7 patients with cirrhosis in the 24-week group achieving SVR. An additional option that has been recommended for patients who previously failed therapy for genotype 4 is peginterferon, ribavirin, and sofosbuvir for 12 weeks, which in 28 naive patients achieved an SVR rate of 96% in the phase 3 Neutrino study, although the only patient who relapsed had cirrhosis.[10] To date, there are no reports prospectively assessing the efficacy of this regimen in cirrhotic nonresponders.

GENOTYPES 5 AND 6

The treatment of cirrhotic patients with genotypes 5 and 6 is based on expert opinion with minimal data. The current recommendation for all genotype 5 patients, including those with cirrhosis, is triple therapy with peginterferon, ribavirin, and sofosbuvir 400 mg for genotype 5. This recommendation is based on a single patient without cirrhosis who received peginterferon, ribavirin, and sofosbuvir and achieved SVR,

Table 6
On-treatment monitoring: genotype 2 with cirrhosis

Treatment Week	1	2	4	8	12	16[a]/EOT	SVR 12
CBC	X[a]	X[a]	X	X	X	X	—
Creatinine	—	—	X	X	X	X	—
Calculated GFR	—	—	X	X	X	X	—
Hepatic fxn panel	—	—	X	X	X	X	—
TSH (with IFN)	—	—	—	—	X	—	—
HCV RNA	—	—	X	—	X	—	X

Sixteen weeks is the preferred duration in patients with cirrhosis regardless of treatment status.

Safety data from phase II/III studies suggest that no difference in monitoring is required for patients with Child A cirrhosis.

[a] Consider CBC at weeks 1 and 2 if using ribavirin with Hgb level less than 12 g/dL or GFR less than 60 mL/min.

Table 7
On-treatment monitoring: genotype 3 with cirrhosis for sofosbuvir plus RBV for 24 weeks

Treatment Week	1	2	4	8	12	16	20	24/EOT	SVR 12
CBC	X[a]	X[a]	X	X	X	X	X	X	—
Creatinine	—	—	X	X	X	X	X	X	—
Calculated GFR	—	—	X	X	X	X	X	X	—
Hepatic fxn panel	—	—	X	X	X	X	X	X	—
TSH (with IFN)	—	—	—	—	X	—	—	X	—
HCV RNA	—	—	X	—	X	—	—	X	X

Safety data from phase II/III studies suggest that no difference in monitoring is required for patients with Child A cirrhosis.

[a] Consider CBC at weeks 1 and 2 if using ribavirin with Hgb level less than 12 g/dL or GFR less than 60 mL/min.

and more studies are required in this population genotype.[10] For genotype 6, there are limited data in cirrhotic patients, but sofosbuvir and ledipasvir for 12 weeks is the recommended therapy. This recommendation is based on a small study that examined 25 patients (92% treatment naive and Asian, of whom 2 of 25 [8%] had cirrhosis), all of whom achieved SVR except for 1 patient who experienced relapse and who had discontinued therapy at treatment week 8.[27] There are no other data with DAAs other than peginterferon, ribavirin, and sofosbuvir in the phase 3 Neutrino study. All 6 patients with genotype 6 achieved SVR. Targeted studies are required.

The monitoring of patients with cirrhosis depends on the use of ribavirin. Sample monitoring is shown in **Tables 5–7**. Patients with cirrhosis who are on ribavirin-based therapy should receive a complete blood count (CBC) at weeks 0, 1, 2, and 4 in the first month, and, for those who are not on ribavirin therapies, CBC should be monitored monthly and at weeks 12 and 24 if extending therapy for this duration. Drug-drug interaction should also be assessed because those with cirrhosis are not able to tolerate acute on chronic liver failure well, although all of the medicines listed here have been shown to be safe in large studies with compensated cirrhosis.

In summary, it is now the expectation that patients with compensated cirrhosis will achieve SVR rates similar to those who do not have cirrhosis. The most significant population requiring new therapies is the genotype 3 treatment-experienced cirrhotic patients, in whom the optimal therapy remains unclear. Once SVR is achieved, patients should continue to be monitored for complications, including varices decompensation, and hepatocellular carcinoma.

REFERENCES

1. Alter MJ. Epidemiology of hepatitis C virus infection. World J Gastroenterol 2007; 13(17):2436–41.
2. Chak E, Talal AH, Sherman KE, et al. Hepatitis C virus infection in USA: an estimate of true prevalence. Liver Int 2011;31(8):1090–101.
3. Davis GL, Alter MJ, El-Serag H, et al. Aging of hepatitis C virus (HCV)-infected persons in the United States: a multiple cohort model of HCV prevalence and disease progression. Gastroenterology 2010;138(2):513–21, 521.e1–6.
4. Razavi H, Elkhoury AC, Elbasha E, et al. Chronic hepatitis C virus (HCV) disease burden and cost in the United States. Hepatology 2013;57(6):2164–70.
5. Schuppan D, Afdhal NH. Liver cirrhosis. Lancet 2008;371(9615):838–51.

6. Bruix J, Sherman M. Management of hepatocellular carcinoma: an update. Hepatology 2011;53(3):1020–2.
7. Garcia-Tsao G, Sanyal AJ, Grace ND, et al. Prevention and management of gastroesophageal varices and variceal hemorrhage in cirrhosis. Hepatology 2007;46(3):922–38.
8. Jacobson I, et al. SVR results of a once-daily regimen of simeprevir (TMC435) plus sofosbuvir (GS-7977) with or without ribavirin in cirrhotic and non-cirrhotic HCV genotype 1 treatment-naive and prior null responder patients: The COSMOS study. In the 64th annual meeting of the American Association for the Study of Liver Diseases (AASLD 2013). 2013.
9. Zeuzem S, Dusheiko GM, Salupere R, et al. Sofosbuvir and ribavirin in HCV genotypes 2 and 3. N Engl J Med 2014;370(21):1993–2001.
10. Lawitz E, Mangia A, Wyles D, et al. Sofosbuvir for previously untreated chronic hepatitis C infection. N Engl J Med 2013;368(20):1878–87.
11. Lawitz E, Sulkowski MS, Ghalib R, et al. Simeprevir plus sofosbuvir, with or without ribavirin, to treat chronic infection with hepatitis C virus genotype 1 in non-responders to pegylated interferon and ribavirin and treatment-naive patients: the COSMOS randomised study. Lancet 2014;384(9956):1756–65.
12. Bacon BR, Gordon SC, Lawitz E, et al. Boceprevir for previously treated chronic HCV genotype 1 infection. N Engl J Med 2011;364(13):1207–17.
13. Jacobson IM, McHutchison JG, Dusheiko G, et al. Telaprevir for previously untreated chronic hepatitis C virus infection. N Engl J Med 2011;364(25):2405–16.
14. McHutchison JG, Lawitz EJ, Shiffman ML, et al. Peginterferon alfa-2b or alfa-2a with ribavirin for treatment of hepatitis C infection. N Engl J Med 2009;361(6):580–93.
15. van der Meer AJ, Veldt BJ, Feld JJ, et al. Association between sustained virological response and all-cause mortality among patients with chronic hepatitis C and advanced hepatic fibrosis. JAMA 2012;308(24):2584–93.
16. Afdhal N, Zeuzem S, Kwo P, et al. Ledipasvir and sofosbuvir for untreated HCV genotype 1 infection. N Engl J Med 2014;370(20):1889–98.
17. Poordad F, Hezode C, Trinh R, et al. ABT-450/r-ombitasvir and dasabuvir with ribavirin for hepatitis C with cirrhosis. N Engl J Med 2014;370(21):1973–82.
18. Afdhal N, Reddy KR, Nelson DR, et al. Ledipasvir and sofosbuvir for previously treated HCV genotype 1 infection. N Engl J Med 2014;370(16):1483–93.
19. Yin J, Li N, Han Y, et al. Effect of antiviral treatment with nucleotide/nucleoside analogs on postoperative prognosis of hepatitis B virus-related hepatocellular carcinoma: a two-stage longitudinal clinical study. J Clin Oncol 2013;31(29):3647–55.
20. Wyles DL, Pockros PJ, Yang JC, et al. Retreatment of patients who failed prior sofosbuvir-based regimens with all oral fixed-dose combination ledipasvir/sofosbuvir plus ribavirin for 12 weeks. Hepatology 2014;60(S):235.
21. European Association for Study of Liver, European Organisation for Research and Treatment of Cancer. EASL-EORTC clinical practice guidelines: management of hepatocellular carcinoma. Eur J Cancer 2012;48(5):599–641.
22. Jacobson IM, Gordon SC, Kowdley KV, et al. Sofosbuvir for hepatitis C genotype 2 or 3 in patients without treatment options. N Engl J Med 2013;368(20):1867–77.
23. Kamal SM, El Tawil AA, Nakano T, et al. Peginterferon α-2b and ribavirin therapy in chronic hepatitis C genotype 4: impact of treatment duration and viral kinetics on sustained virological response. Gut 2005;54(6):858–66.
24. Stanislas P, Reddy KR, Hezode C, et al. Interferon-free regimens of ombitasvir and ABT-450/r with or without ribavirin in patients with HCV genotype 4 infection: PEARL-I study results. Hepatology 2014;60(S1):1928.

25. Rama K, Kohli A, Sidharthan S, et al. Treatment of hepatitis C genotype 4 with ledipasvir and sofosbuvir for 12 weeks: results of the SYNERGY trial. Hepatology 2014;60(S1):240.

26. Ruane PJ, Ain D, Stryker R, et al. Sofosbuvir plus ribavirin for the treatment of chronic genotype 4 hepatitis C virus infection in patients of Egyptian ancestry. J Hepatol 2015;62(5):1040–6.

27. Gane EJ, Hyland RH, An D, et al. High efficacy of LDV/SOF regimens for 12 weeks for patients with HCV genotype 3 or 6 infection. Hepatology 2014; 60(Late Breaking Abstracts):1274.

Current Management of Hepatitis C Virus

Regimens for Peri-Liver Transplant Patients

Varun Saxena, MD, MS, Norah Terrault, MD, MPH*

KEYWORDS

- Hepatitis C virus • Liver transplant • Direct-acting antivirals
- Recurrent hepatitis C virus • Sofosbuvir • Simeprevir • Ledipasvir
- Cholestatic hepatitis

KEY POINTS

- The primary goal of hepatitis C virus treatment in the peri-liver transplant setting is to prevent liver-related complications and graft loss caused by recurrence of hepatitis C virus after liver transplant.
- Approved direct-acting antivirals against hepatitis C offer a safe and effective option for treatment in the peri-liver transplant period with primary determinants of use guided by renal and liver function.
- Hepatitis C virus treatment in patients with decompensated cirrhosis with newer direct-acting antivirals are generally well tolerated and provide cure rates ranging from 50% to 94%.
- On-treatment virologic responses with newer direct-acting antivirals are almost universal providing the opportunity to treat to achieve at least 4 weeks viral negativity before liver transplant.

INTRODUCTION

The World Health Organization estimates that about 3% of the world's population has been infected with hepatitis C virus (HCV) and that there are more than 170 million with chronic disease who are at risk of developing liver cirrhosis and/or liver cancer.[1] The

Dr V. Saxena has nothing to disclose. Dr N. Terrault discloses research support from Gilead, Genetech/Roche, Vertex, Novartis, Eisai, and AbbVie and has served as consultant for Bristol-Myers Squibb.
Division of Gastroenterology and Hepatology, Department of Medicine, University of California, San Francisco, San Francisco, CA, USA
* Corresponding author. University of California, San Francisco, Box 0538, 513 Parnassus Avenue, S357, San Francisco, CA 94143.
E-mail address: norah.terrault@ucsf.edu

Clin Liver Dis 19 (2015) 669–688
http://dx.doi.org/10.1016/j.cld.2015.06.007
1089-3261/15/$ – see front matter © 2015 Elsevier Inc. All rights reserved.

prevalence of chronic HCV infection in the United States has been estimated at 2.7 million persons per the most recent National Health and Nutrition Examination Survey (NHANES) data,[2] but a study accounting for high-risk groups underrepresented in NHANES suggested a US prevalence of 5.2 million.[3] Given this burden of disease, is it not surprising that HCV infection remains the most common indication for liver transplant (LT) in the United States.[4]

Recurrence of HCV after LT is universal in viremic patients undergoing LT; in adjusted models, recurrent HCV leads to an approximately 28% (95% confidence interval [CI]: 15%–40%) increase in graft loss and a 17% (95% CI: 3%–32%) increase in recipient mortality compared with LT recipients without HCV.[5] The natural history of recurrent HCV is significantly more aggressive compared with the natural history before LT, with 20% to 54% developing bridging fibrosis/cirrhosis at 5 years[6] and 2% to 9% developing the aggressive and rapidly progressive fibrosing cholestatic HCV within 1 year after LT.[7] On the other hand, successful HCV eradication either before LT or after LT has been shown to improve post-LT outcomes[8] and, therefore, is the goal of HCV treatment in the peri-LT setting.

The development of direct-acting antivirals (DAAs) against HCV has revolutionized the treatment of HCV (**Table 1**). The first 2 DAAs included the first-generation NS3/4A protease inhibitors (PIs), telaprevir and boceprevir, which were approved by the US Food and Drug Administration (FDA) in 2011 for use in combination with peginterferon (PEG-IFN) and ribavirin (RBV) to treat chronic genotype 1 HCV. With the approval of second-generation NS3/4A PIs and additional DAAs, the first-generation PIs are no longer used in the United States. Simeprevir (SMV), a second-generation PI, was FDA approved for use in combination with PEG-IFN and RBV for genotype 1 HCV in November 2013. Soon thereafter, the first-in-class nucleotide NS5B polymerase inhibitor sofosbuvir (SOF) was FDA approved in December 2013 with pan-genotypic activity. More recently, the FDA approved the fixed-dose combination of ledipasvir (LDV), a NS5A replication complex inhibitor, and SOF in October 2014. This approval was followed closely by the FDA approval of combined ombitasvir (OBV) (an NS5A replication complex inhibitor) and ritonavir (r) boosted paritaprevir (PTV) (a PI), copackaged with dasabuvir (DBV) (the only approved non-nucleoside NS5B polymerase inhibitor) (OBV-PTV-r/DBV). Although not yet approved by the FDA, daclatasvir (DCV), another NS5A inhibitor, was approved in Europe in August 2014 and is anticipated to gain approval in the United States in 2015. With the availability of these and future DAAs (see **Table 1**), the era of interferon-containing HCV treatment regimens for peri-LT patients is over.

Management of HCV in the peri-LT setting uses several different strategies (**Fig. 1**). Wait-listed patients can be treated with the goal of achieving pre-LT cure and/or preventing HCV recurrence after LT. In the post-LT setting, HCV treatment can be used either preemptively in the early post-LT period to prevent clinically significant disease or used for patients with established recurrent disease, including those with cirrhosis who have failed prior therapies, all with the intent to achieve cure. In the pre-DAA era when PEG-IFN and RBV were the mainstays for treating HCV, the dominant strategy used was the treatment of post-LT patients who showed evidence of severe or progressive recurrent disease.[9] This approach reflected the diminished tolerability of PEG-IFN and RBV and low rate of sustained virologic response (SVR). Although the addition of first-generation PIs, telaprevir and boceprevir, improved efficacy significantly, the poor tolerability of therapy remained a significant barrier. In contrast, current DAA combination therapies are well tolerated, allowing a broader array of peri-LT patients to be considered for therapy and provide new opportunities to both prevent and treat recurrent HCV disease with high efficacy.

Table 1
Characteristics of new DAAs against HCV

DAA	Mechanism of Action	Genotypic Coverage	Special Considerations
Approved			
Telaprevir	NS3/4A protease inhibitor	1	Discontinued in United States
Boceprevir	NS3/4A protease inhibitor	1	To be discontinued in United States December 2015
Simeprevir	NS3/4A protease inhibitor	1, 4	Mild CYP3A inhibition Indirect hyperbilirubinemia
Sofosbuvir	Nucleotide NS5B polymerase inhibitor	Pan-genotypic	Renal clearance
Ledipasvir	NS5A replication complex inhibitor	Pan-genotypic	—
Paritaprevir/ ritonavir	NS3/4A protease inhibitor	1, 4	CYP3A inhibition Indirect hyperbilirubinemia
Ombitasvir	NS5A replication complex inhibitor	1, 4	—
Dasabuvir	Non-nucleoside NS5B polymerase inhibitor	1, 4	—
Experimental			
Asunaprevir	NS3/4A protease inhibitor	1, 4	Weak CYP3A induction
Grazoprevir	NS3/4A protease inhibitor	Pan-genotypic	—
Daclatasvir	NS5A replication complex inhibitor	Pan-genotypic	—
GS-5816	NS5A replication complex inhibitor	Pan-genotypic	—
Elbasvir	NS5A replication complex inhibitor	Pan-genotypic	—
Beclabuvir	Non-nucleoside NS5B polymerase inhibitor	1	—

HEPATITIS C VIRUS TREATMENT BEFORE LIVER TRANSPLANT TO ACHIEVE CURE

In general, patients with indications for LT have decompensated cirrhosis. However, patients with hepatocellular carcinoma (HCC) may have compensated cirrhosis. These latter patients can be treated for cure using the same guiding principles as applied to patients who are not wait-listed for LT (see the article by Paul Kwo elsewhere in this issue). Moreover, because patients with HCC garner exception points that ensure that all patients whose HCC remains within the Milan criteria have access to LT, these patients are ideal patients to treat with DAA combinations before LT with the goal of achieving cure *and* preventing post-LT recurrence (see section *Hepatitis C virus treatment before liver transplant to prevent hepatitis C virus recurrence*).

For patients with decompensated cirrhosis, the decision to treat for cure is a more complex one. Certainly, there are now DAA combinations that are safe and can offer cure to this previously largely incurable group. Potential gains from achieving cure in patients with decompensated cirrhosis include a reversal of complications of cirrhosis, improved quality of life, reduced risk of wait-list mortality, and prevention

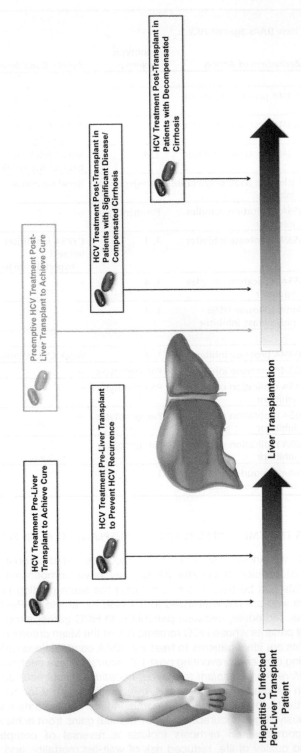

Fig. 1. HCV treatment strategies for peri-LT patients.

of HCV recurrence after LT (if LT occurs). Most of these potential gains are still theoretic, as long-term studies of outcomes in patients with decompensated cirrhosis are lacking. Moreover, there may be a potential downside of treating patients with decompensated cirrhosis on the wait-list, in that model of end-stage liver disease (MELD) scores may decrease with virologic cure, making LT less likely, but not improving the complications of liver disease sufficiently to make avoidance of LT desirable.

The HCV therapies currently approved in the United States for use in patients with decompensated cirrhosis included SOF/RBV, LDV/SOF with or without RBV, and SMV/SOF (patients with Child-Pugh [CP] class B cirrhosis only). OBV-PTV-r/DBV with or without RBV is not an option. SOF is extensively metabolized in the liver to the pharmacologically active metabolite GS-461203 with eventual dephosphorylation to the inactive metabolite GS-331007.[10] Relative to patients with normal hepatic function, the GS-331007 areas under the curves from 0 to 24 hours ($AUCs_{0-24}$) are 18% and 9% greater in patients with CP class B and C cirrhosis, respectively; no dose adjustments for SOF are needed for patients with advanced cirrhosis.[10] Renal clearance is the major elimination pathway for SOF, via GS-331007; compared with those with normal renal function, SOF $AUC_{0-\infty}$ was 1.7-fold higher and the GS-331007 $AUC_{0-\infty}$ was 4.5-fold higher in those with an estimated glomerular filtration rate (eGFR) less than 30 mL/min/1.73 m^2.[10] Consequently, SOF is not recommended for patients with an eGFR less than 30 mL/min/1.73 m^2.[10] No pharmacokinetic data are available to guide dosing in patients with combined liver and renal dysfunction, a frequent clinical scenario in patients with advanced decompensated cirrhosis.

SMV is extensively metabolized by the hepatic cytochrome CYP3A system and eliminated via biliary excretion.[11] Relative to patients with normal hepatic function, SMV AUC_{0-24} values are 2.4-fold and 5.2-fold higher in patients with CP class B and class C cirrhosis, respectively.[12] Higher exposure to SMV has been associated with increased frequency of adverse reactions in clinical trials.[11] As a result, the risks and benefits of SMV use need to be carefully considered in patients with CP class B cirrhosis and avoided in patients with CP class C cirrhosis.[11]

The safety and efficacy of SMV plus SOF in patients with decompensated cirrhosis have been evaluated is real-life cohorts. In a national study of 156 patients (101 with CP class A cirrhosis, 49 with CP class B cirrhosis, and 6 CP class C cirrhosis) treated for 12 weeks with SMV/SOF with (35%) and without (65%) RBV,[13] patients with CP class B or C cirrhosis (vs patients with CP class A cirrhosis) developed further hepatic decompensation more frequently (20% vs 3%; P value less than .01) (Table 2) while achieving SVR at 12 weeks after treatment discontinuation (SVR12) less frequently than patients with CP class A cirrhosis (73% vs 91%, P value less than .01) (Fig. 2).[13] Similar SVR12 results were reported with compensated and decompensated cirrhosis in the HCV-TARGET cohort (87% and 75%, respectively).[14] Among those with a baseline MELD score greater than 10, HCV-TARGET reported an SVR12 rate of 74% (79 of 107) among those receiving SMV/SOF and 66% (19 of 29) among those receiving SMV/SOF and RBV.[15] In terms of safety and tolerability, a recent case report suggested SMV/SOF may be associated with worsening hepatic decompensation in patients with CP class C cirrhosis.[16] However, in a controlled study, patients with decompensated cirrhosis treated with SMV/SOF had a similar frequency of hepatic decompensation during treatment to matched controls followed for a similar duration of time (9% vs 10%, P = .78),[13] suggesting safety events during treatment may reflect the natural history of decompensated cirrhosis. The complexity of establishing a causal relationship between drug exposures and decompensating events in patients with advanced cirrhosis is well recognized.[17]

Table 2
Safety outcomes by HCV treatment regimen in patients with decompensated cirrhosis

Regimen	N	Safety Outcomes
SMV/SOF ± RBV × 12 wk[13]	49 CP class B; 6 CP class C	• 11% (6 of 55) early treatment discontinuation • 22% (12 of 55) hospitalized • 20% (11 of 55) infection requiring antibiotics • 20% (11 of 55) further hepatic decompensation • 2% (1 of 55) death
LDV/SOF + RBV × 12–24 wk[18]	59 CP class B; 49 CP class C	• CP and MELD scores improved from baseline in most patients • Low rates of grade 3/4 AEs, serious AEs (more common in 24-wk arm) • No treatment discontinuations in 12-wk arm, 3 in 24-wk arm • 5% (3 of 59) deaths in CP class B, 6% (3 of 49) deaths in CP class C, none attributed to study drugs
LDV/SOF + RBV × 24 wk[19]	13 CP class B	• 2 patients experienced serious AEs: one caused by patient's baseline bipolar disorder and one caused by anemia, chest pain, and cholecystitis • No deaths
SOF/RBV[15]	88 Cirrhosis and MELD >10	• 31% (27 of 88) had a serious AE, 11% (10 of 88) had hepatic decompensation*, 8% (7 of 88) had infections • No deaths
SOF/RBV × 24 wk[24]	15 CP class B; 1 CP class C	• Mean change from baseline of albumin was 0.4 g/dL, of bilirubin was −0.2 mg/dL, and of MELD score was −1 • Improvement of baseline ascites and hepatic encephalopathy
SOF/DCV + RBV × 12 wk[26]	12 CP class A; 32 CP class B; 16 CP class C	• 17% (10 of 60) with serious AEs, all considered unrelated to study treatment • 18% (11 of 60) with grade 3/4 AEs: 4 related to study treatment (anemia, noncardiac chest pain, arthralgia, headache) • 2% (1 of 60) discontinued because of AE: discontinued at time of transplant (attained pTVR) • No deaths

Abbreviations: AE, adverse event; pTVR, post-LT virologic response.
 * Combined pre-LT and post-LT patients.

In contrast to the pharmacokinetic data for SMV or SOF, the pharmacokinetic data for LDV in subjects with severe renal (eGFR <30 mL/min/m³) or hepatic (CP class C cirrhosis) impairment suggest no significant differences compared with healthy subjects.[18] Furthermore, safety data are reassuring for use of LDV/SOF in patients with decompensated cirrhosis.[19,20] In the US study of LDV/SOF with RBV (escalating doses starting at 600 mg/d) in 59 patients with CP class B cirrhosis and 49 patients with CP class C cirrhosis (SOLAR-1), SVR12 was achieved in 45 of 52 (87%) patients treated for 12 weeks and 42 of 47 (89%) patients treated for 24 weeks (see **Fig. 2**).[19] In a similar study from Europe (SOLAR-2), LDV/SOF with RBV resulted in SVR12 rates of 86% (37 of 43) versus 85% (35 of 41) in genotype 1 patients with CP class B/C cirrhosis treated for 12 weeks versus 24 weeks (see **Fig. 2**).[21] Serious treatment-related adverse events (AEs) were rare. In the SOLAR-1 study, treatment

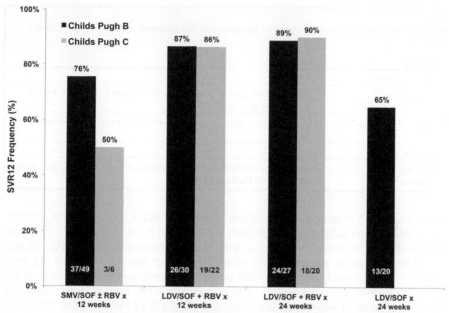

Fig. 2. Virologic responses with varying regimens in patients with decompensated cirrhosis.

was discontinued early because of AEs in 3 patients, and 6 patients died (4 septic shock, 1 renal failure, 1 cardiac arrest) (see **Table 2**). Seven patients underwent LT during the study period and were not included in the analysis: one patient died 2 weeks after LT, and 6 achieved a post-transplant virologic response.[19] In a smaller study of 20 SOF treatment-experienced patients retreated with LDV/SOF without RBV, 13 (65%) with CP class B cirrhosis achieved SVR12 after 12 weeks of treatment and 7 relapsed (see **Fig. 2**).[20] No patients died, and only 2 patients experienced serious AEs: one related to a patient's baseline bipolar disorder and one caused by anemia, chest pain, and cholecystitis (see **Table 2**).[20] Differences in reported SVR rates between these studies may reflect both the patient populations and the use of RBV. Based on data from patients with compensated cirrhosis,[22] the recommended approach to patients with CP class B/C cirrhosis treated with LDV/SOF is to treat for 24 weeks if RBV is not included and 12 weeks if RBV is included (**Table 3**).

SOF/RBV was the first all-oral therapy available to treat patients with decompensated cirrhosis and is currently the only treatment approved for genotypes 2 and 3. Real-world data involving patients with cirrhosis and baseline MELD scores greater than 10 from HCV-TARGET show an SVR12 rate of 81% (21 of 26) among genotype 2–infected patients and a rate of 39% (10 of 26) among genotype 3–infected patients.[15] Among 88 patients with cirrhosis and a baseline MELD score greater than 10 treated with SOF/RBV, 27 (31%) had a serious AE and 10 (11%) had hepatic decompensation, but no patients died.[15] For non–genotype 2 or 3 patients, alternative DAA combinations are available for treatment of patients with decompensated cirrhosis and are preferred over SOF/RBV (see **Table 3**).

Although currently not FDA approved, DCV has been used in Europe in combination with other DAAs in the treatment of HCV. In vitro studies demonstrate that DCV is a substrate of CYP3A, with CYP3A4 the major cytochrome P isoform responsible for

Table 3
Recommended interferon-free regimens by genotype for patients with decompensated cirrhosis

Regimen	Comment
Genotype 1 or 4:	
LDV/SOF + RBV × 12 wk[18]	87% (26 of 30) SVR in patients with CP class B, 86% (19 of 22) SVR in patients with CP class C
LDV/SOF × 24 wk[20]	RBV intolerant; data in patients with decompensated cirrhosis lacking
Genotype 2 or 3:	
SOF/RBV up to 48 wk[39]	Data in patients with decompensated cirrhosis lacking, and exact duration of therapy unknown

the metabolism.[23] Pharmacokinetic studies show the $AUCs_{0-24}$ are 42.7%, 37.6%, and 51.2% lower in subjects with CP class A, CP class B, and CP class C cirrhosis, respectively.[23] In addition, the AUC_{0-24} of DCV was estimated to be 26.4%, 59.8%, and 79.6% higher in subjects with eGFR values of 60, 30, and 15 mL/min/1.73 m^2.[23] In the French compassionate access program, genotype 3–infected patients with cirrhosis (compensated and decompensated) treated with SOF/DCV (±RBV) for 12 and 24 weeks, achieved SVR4 in 76% (22 of 29) and 88% (52 of 59), respectively.[24] In the National Health Service of England real-life experience treating 171 patients with genotype 1 and 3 cirrhosis (61% and 69% CP class B, 8% and 13% CP class C, respectively) with SOF/DCV (±RBV) for 12 weeks, the SVR12 rates were 80% for genotype 1 and 70% for genotype 3.[25] The ALLY-1 trial examining a 12-week regimen of SOF/DCV with RBV (initial dose of 600 mg/d, adjusted to 1000 mg/d based on hemoglobin levels and creatinine clearance) in a predominantly genotype 1–infected population (genotype 1a: 57%, genotype 1b: 18%) resulted in SVR12 rates of 94% (30 of 32) and 56% (9 of 16) in patients with CP class B and CP class C cirrhosis, respectively (see **Fig. 2**).[26] Serious AEs occurred in 11 of 60 (17%) patients with cirrhosis, none related to study treatment; there were no deaths (see **Table 2**).[26] For patients with decompensated cirrhosis in the United States, the future availability of DCV will provide more treatment options for genotype 3–infected patients and additional treatment options for genotype 1– or genotype 4–infected patients.

In a small number of patients with *compensated* cirrhosis who achieved HCV cure with older therapies, liver histology has been shown to improve.[27,28] There is hope that achieving HCV cure in patients with *decompensated* cirrhosis may halt progression of decompensating events and prevent LT. Among 129 HCV-infected patients with decompensated cirrhosis treated with PEG-IFN and RBV, decompensation events occurred in 88% (52 of 59) of the untreated control group, 69% (33 of 48) of the non-SVR group, and 23% (3 of 13) of the SVR group, suggesting a protective effect of cure.[29] Among SOF/LDV-treated patients, the median (range) changes in the CP and MELD scores from baseline to 4 weeks post treatment were −1 (−3 to 2) and −1 (−5 to 10), respectively, among patients with baseline CP class B cirrhosis and was −1 (−3 to 0) and −1 (−6 to 2), respectively, among patients with baseline CP class C cirrhosis.[19] Among patients treated for 24 weeks with SOF/RBV, the mean change from baseline of albumin was 0.4 g/dL, of bilirubin was −0.2 mg/dL, and of MELD score was −1; some patients showed improvement in ascites and hepatic encephalopathy (see **Table 2**).[30] As most studies with DAA combination therapy have evaluated MELD and clinical benefits at SVR12, longer-term follow-up studies are necessary to determine the benefits of HCV cure among patients with decompensated cirrhosis.

HEPATITIS C VIRUS TREATMENT BEFORE LIVER TRANSPLANT TO PREVENT HEPATITIS C VIRUS RECURRENCE

For patients who achieve SVR before LT, 100% are HCV free after LT.[31] However, a shorter treatment course aimed at achieving an undetectable HCV RNA at the time of LT (rather than SVR) can significantly reduce the risk of post-LT HCV recurrence.[32–38] This HCV treatment strategy may be especially useful in patients whose time of LT is predictable, such as living-donor LT recipients or those with HCC. This strategy was first established in the Adult-to-Adult Living Donor Liver Transplantation Cohort Study,[36] with patients randomized to a low accelerating dose regimen of PEG-IFN and RBV or observation before LT.[36] The outcome of interest was achieving post-LT virologic response (pTVR) that was defined as an undetectable HCV RNA 12 weeks after LT.[36] Forty-four treated patients underwent LT of which 26 (59%) achieved an undetectable HCV RNA by the time of LT and 11 (25%) achieved pTVR.[36] Importantly, those who were treated for less than 8 weeks, 8 to 16 weeks, or greater than 16 weeks achieved pTVR at 0%, 18%, and 50%, respectively.[36] Despite not directly evaluating the duration of HCV RNA negativity as a predictor of pTVR, this study shows that HCV treatment before LT can prevent HCV recurrence and that duration of therapy (and, therefore, likely the duration of HCV RNA undetectability before LT) was an important predictor of treatment success.[36] With the first-generation PI (telaprevir or boceprevir)-based triple therapy, an improved on-treatment response was seen but offset by the high frequency of treatment-associated AEs.[39,40]

With the availability of the newer DAAs, PEG-IFN no longer has any role in pre-LT antiviral therapy aimed to prevent post-LT HCV recurrence. DAA combinations achieve nearly universal on-treatment virologic responses.[41–43] The time to and duration of HCV RNA negativity are critical elements of using this antiviral strategy to prevent HCV recurrence after LT. The factors potentially influencing the virologic responses on treatment include the severity of cirrhosis, prior treatment experience, and the DAA combination used. The landmark study was a phase 2 pilot study of SOF and weight-based RBV in 61 patients infected with genotypes 1 to 4 and a CP score of 7 or less listed for LT accruing a MELD exception point for HCC.[44] On an intent-to-treat basis, 59% of patients initiating therapy achieved pTVR. However, of the 43 patients who were treated *and* had an undetectable HCV RNA at the time of LT, 30 (70%) achieved pTVR.[44] The duration of continuously undetectable HCV RNA was associated with the likelihood of achieving pTVR, with only 1 of 26 patients with continuously undetectable HCV RNA for at least 30 days before LT developing recurrent HCV.[44] Safety events in this study occurred at similar frequency to what was observed in the registration trials for SOF and weight-based RBV. As a result of this study, SOF and weight-based RBV is FDA approved for patients with HCC awaiting LT with available data supporting a minimum of 4 weeks of HCV RNA negativity before LT to maximize the chance of pTVR.[45]

Available data highlight the heterogeneity of the on-treatment virologic responses. In a study of 25 genotype 1 to 4 HCV–infected patients with CP class A and B cirrhosis and portal hypertension (hepatic venous pressure gradient >6 mm Hg) treated with SOF and RBV,[30] 75% of patients with decompensated cirrhosis achieved an undetectable HCV RNA level by week 4 of treatment (**Fig. 3**).[30] In a study of 55 patients with decompensated cirrhosis treated with SMV/SOF with or without RBV, 62% achieved an on-treatment response by 4 weeks (see **Fig. 3**), with a median time to undetectable viral load of 32 days.[13] Among 20 patients with CP class B cirrhosis who underwent LDV/SOF, 75% achieved a negative viral load at treatment week 4% and 100% by week 12 (see **Fig. 3**).[20] Based on these data, the goal should be to initiate

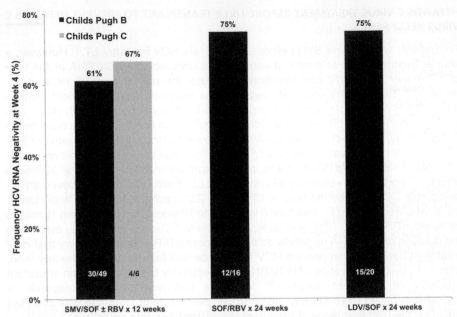

Fig. 3. On-treatment virologic response at week 4 with varying regimens in patients with decompensated cirrhosis.

treatment at least 6 to 10 weeks before LT in order to achieve approximately 4 weeks of HCV RNA negativity before LT and to maximize the likelihood of achieving pTVR.

For patients with compensated cirrhosis, several treatment options exist; but for decompensated cirrhosis, LDV/SOF with/without RBV (genotype 1, 4, and 6) and, until DCV becomes available, SOF and RBV dual therapy (genotypes 2 and 3) should be considered. The treatment duration should be timed to LT if possible, and this is most easily accomplished in patients with living donors or those with exception status (eg, HCC). Because the cost of treatment is closely tied with the duration of therapy, it remains to be determined whether treatment for prevention (with a possibly shorter duration of treatment) is more cost-effective than treatment post-LT.

PREEMPTIVE HEPATITIS C VIRUS TREATMENT AFTER LIVER TRANSPLANT TO ACHIEVE CURE

The preemptive strategy initiates HCV therapy in the immediate or early posttransplant period, before the development of recurrent disease. This therapeutic approach is predicated on the knowledge that HCV viremia rapidly declines with removal of the recipient's cirrhotic liver and increases gradually in the hours to days following LT.[46] Potent DAAs against HCV given immediately at the time of LT, along with removal of the infected organ, may avoid the rapid recurrence of viremia and also allow for shorter and, thus, more cost-effective HCV management. However, the safety and efficacy of DAAs in the immediate transplant period are unknown; the benefits of preemptive versus delayed posttransplant therapy remain to be established. Currently, the CRUSH-C consortium is examining the safety and efficacy of LDV/SOF administered in patients infected with chronic genotype 1 or 4 HCV in the perioperative LT setting (ClinicalTrials.gov NCT02350569).

Another preemptive strategy is to use adjuvant antibody therapy in patients who are on antiviral therapy at the time of LT. In a phase 3, open-label randomized study, 84 HCV-infected wait-listed patients receiving DAAs leading up to transplant were randomized 1:1:1 to hepatitis C immunoglobulin (HCIG) 200 mg/kg, 300 mg/kg, or observation.[47] In preliminary data, 63 patients were treated pre-LT with DAA-based therapy for a median of 63 days with post-transplant reinfection occurring in 1/21 (5%) in the 300 mg/kg, 7/22 (32%) in 200 mg/kg group and 6/20 (30%) controls.[47] These preliminary results suggest use of higher dose HCIG may be beneficial as an adjuvant therapy for patients on HCV therapy undergoing LT.

HEPATITIS C VIRUS TREATMENT AFTER LIVER TRANSPLANT TO ACHIEVE CURE

Achievement of SVR after LT is associated with improved graft and patient survival[48] and is the goal of every LT recipient. Prior treatment guidelines recommended antiviral therapy be initiated after LT only if there is moderate fibrosis ($\geq$F2 on a scale of 4), moderate or severe necroinflammatory activity ($\geq$A3 on scale of 4), or cholestatic hepatitis.[9] Post-LT therapy with PEG-IFN and RBV, started within the first 6 months after LT and before the presence of fibrosis on protocol biopsies, was no more effective than delaying treatment until disease progression was present.[49] However, with the improved safety profiles of IFN-free therapies, earlier post-LT therapy may be merited to gain full survival benefit from cure and decrease the cost related to monitoring and management of recurrent disease complications.

Significant Fibrosis/Compensated Cirrhosis

SVR rates with PEG-IFN and RBV were approximately 30% for genotype 1 and 60% to 75% for non-1 genotypes.[50] Dose reductions were frequently required, and treatment discontinuation was common; but acute and chronic rejection were infrequent, occurring in 2% and less than 1%, respectively. SVR rates with first-generation PI-based triple therapy were substantially higher with 63% achieving cure.[51] However, tolerability and safety were significant challenges with telaprevir- and boceprevir-based therapy,[51,52] including worsening of renal function in up to 38% of patients.[53] This worsening was possibly related to the degree of anemia or from the result of calcineurin inhibitor toxicity from either altered pharmacokinetics in the setting of CYP3A4/5 inhibition or P-glycoprotein inhibition caused by the PI.[52] Thus, the addition of a DAA substantially increased the success of therapy; however, the side effects of the first-generation PIs plus the need for use of PEG-IFN and RBV resulted in a complex therapy for patients and providers. Although some countries without access to newer DAAs continue to use PI triple therapy with success, in the United States, newer DAA combinations have supplanted its use.

The all-oral antiviral regimens show improved efficacy and safety over the first-generation PI-based triple therapy for LT recipients. In a phase 2 clinical trial, 44 LT recipients with HCV genotypes 1 to 4 who were at least 6 months post-LT received SOF and RBV for 24 weeks.[54] All patients had a CP score of 7 or less and a MELD score of 17 or less, and patients with signs of decompensation were excluded.[54] RBV was started at 400 mg/d and was escalated based on tolerability and degree of anemia.[54] All patients achieved an end-of-treatment response, and 28 (70%) achieved SVR12 (**Fig. 4**). Average RBV doses did not differ between those who did and did not achieve SVR12.[54] Anemia requiring erythropoietin and/or blood transfusions occurred in 20%,[54] more than half of the frequency seen with first-generation PI-based triple therapy.[51,52] Furthermore, there were no deaths, graft losses, or episodes of rejection or any significant drug-drug interactions between SOF and

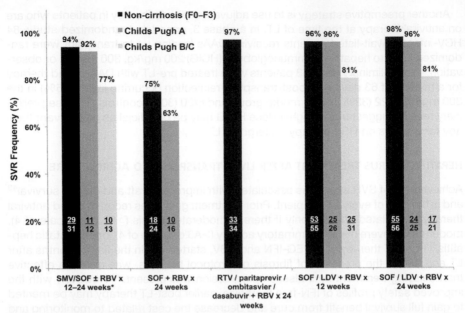

Fig. 4. Virologic responses in post-LT patients with varying regimens by degree of liver disease. [a] CP class A = cirrhosis with a MELD score less than 10; CP class B/C = cirrhosis with a MELD score of 10 or greater. Of note, results for F0-F3 and CP class A LT recipients in the SOLAR-2 study were presented in a combined format but were included in F0-F3 bars.

tacrolimus or cyclosporine.[55] SOF and RBV are currently recommended for post-LT patients with genotype 2 or 3 disease.[45]

Real-world experience with SMV/SOF with or without RBV for genotype 1 LT recipients has been reported. In a study of 123 patients (60% genotype 1A, 30% F3/F4, 80% treatment experienced), SVR12 was achieved in 90%.[56] One patient died of drug-induced lung injury while on treatment.[56] In interim analysis of the HCV-TARGET cohort of 131 LT recipients, 90% achieved SVR4, with 86% SVR4 in those with cirrhosis and 94% in those without.[57] Serious AEs were rare in both studies, and there were no episodes of graft rejection.[56,57] SMV does not seem to have clinically significant interactions with tacrolimus, but cyclosporine increased SMV levels by approximately 6-fold; thus, patients on cyclosporine should not be treated with SMV-containing regimens.[58] SMV/SOF with or without RBV for 12 weeks is one of the recommended regimens for genotype 1–infected LT recipients with compensated liver disease.[45]

LDV/SOF with RBV was evaluated in a phase 2 study of 223 LT recipients with genotype 1 and 4 for 12 or 24 weeks.[19] Fifty percent (n = 111) of the treated patients were without cirrhosis (Metavir fibrosis stage 0–3), 51 (28%) with CP class A cirrhosis, 52 (23%) with CP class B cirrhosis, and 9 (4%) with Child Pugh C cirrhosis.[19] SVR12 was achieved in 96% of F0-F3 patients, 96% with CP class A cirrhosis, and 81% with CP class B/C cirrhosis with SVR rates similar with 12 versus 24 weeks of treatment (see **Fig. 4**).[19] Fatigue, anemia, headache, and nausea were the most common AEs.[19] Seven patients died of causes judged to be unrelated to treatment.[19] In the European SOLAR-2 study of LDV/SOF with RBV in LT recipients, SVR12 was achieved in 95% with F0-3 fibrosis and 98% with compensated CP class A cirrhosis treated for

12 or 24 weeks (no difference by duration of therapy)[21] (see **Fig. 4**).[21] Based on these results, LDV/SOF *with* weight-based RBV for 12 weeks is recommended for LT recipients with compensated and decompensated genotype 1 or 4 HCV disease.[45]

In the CORAL-1 study, 34 LT patients with genotype 1 HCV infection and F0-2 fibrosis were treated with OBV-PTV-r/DBV and RBV for 24 weeks.[59] RBV was dosed at the discretion of the treating physician; 600 to 800 mg/d was the most common dosage at baseline (56%) and at the end of treatment (68%). SVR12 was achieved in 97% (see **Fig. 4**).[59] The one relapse occurred 3 days after treatment discontinuation, and the patient had evidence of NS3, NS5A, and NS5B resistant variants, which were not present at baseline.[59] Serious AEs occurred in 2 patients, and 1 patient discontinued the study drugs because of AEs.[59] Anemia was common and seen in approximately one-third of patients, with 5 patients receiving erythropoietin.[59] Two patients experienced serious AEs: one with hypotension and tachycardia related to tamsulosin administered after elective surgery and one diabetic patient with moderate peripheral edema and pain in extremities.[59] Tacrolimus dosages were modified to 0.5 mg per week or 0.2 mg every 3 days, and cyclosporine dose reductions were to 20% of the pretreated daily dose.[59] No episodes of rejection occurred. Based on these results, OBV-PTV-r/DBV and RBV for 24 weeks is approved for LT recipients with genotype 1 HCV infection with early stage fibrosis ($\leq$F2).[45] A study of this DAA combination in patients with more advanced stages of fibrosis is ongoing (ClinicalTrials.gov NCT01782495).

In the ALLY-1 study, SOF/DCV with RBV for 12 weeks was examined in 53 LT recipients, genotypes 1 and 3, 68% with F0-F3 fibrosis and 30% with CP class A cirrhosis (1 patient missing baseline stage).[26] SVR12 was observed in 50 of 53 (94%). Only 9% experienced serious AEs, and all were unrelated to the study drug.[26] Although SOF/DCV with/without RBV has been used in LT recipients in compassionate access programs,[24,25] efficacy and safety results are not currently available. Coadministration of DCV with cyclosporine or tacrolimus has been investigated in healthy HCV-negative subjects, and DCV did not affect the pharmacokinetics of either calcineurin inhibitor.[60] Although cyclosporine caused a modest increase in DCV exposure with a 40% increase in AUC_{0-24}, dose adjustments for DCV, tacrolimus or cyclosporine are unlikely to be required during coadministration.[60] Availability of DCV in the United States will provide another NS5A inhibitor option for LT recipients, especially those with decompensated cirrhosis.

Decompensated Cirrhosis

In a compassionate access program for LT recipients with severe recurrence and less than 1-year life expectancy, patients with genotype 1 to 4 and decompensated cirrhosis or severe cholestatic hepatitis received variable duration of SOF and RBV with or without PEG-IFN.[61] Only 72 (69%) patients completed 24 to 48 weeks of treatment; 7 discontinuations caused by AEs, 12 repeat LTs, and 13 deaths were reported.[61] Overall, excluding repeat LT and patients without data available, 62% achieved SVR12.[61]

Data using other DAA combinations are more limited. Drawing on real-world experience, 131 genotype 1–infected LT recipients were treated with SMV/SOF with or without RBV for 12 or 24 weeks with SVR4 reported in 77% of patients with cirrhosis and a MELD score of 10 or greater (see **Fig. 4**).[62] In LT recipients treated with LDV/SOF with RBV for 12 or 24 weeks, the SVR12 rates were 84% (CP class B cirrhosis, n = 44) and 63% (CP class C cirrhosis, n = 8) (see **Fig. 4**).[19] Of the 10 patients who did not achieve SVR12, 3 relapsed, 5 died (none thought to be related to treatment), and 1 withdrew consent.[19] Only one patient with decompensated cirrhosis had a treatment-related serious AE (hemolytic anemia), and 3 patients discontinued treatment because of AEs.[19] In the SOLAR-2 study, 35 of 36 (97%) of LT recipients with CP class B cirrhosis and 4 of 6 (67%) of LT recipients with CP class C cirrhosis achieved SVR12 with SVR rates similar with 12 versus 24 weeks of treatment (see **Fig. 4**).[21] The safety and efficacy of SOF and DCV with or without RBV has been studied in compassionate access settings. Among 12 post-LT patients with severe recurrent HCV (3 with severe cholestatic HCV), 9 patients completing 24 weeks of treatment had undetectable HCV RNA at treatment end and 5 patients with follow-up achieved SVR4.[63] During treatment, 3 deaths occurred: one caused by rapidly progressive liver failure, one caused by gastrointestinal bleeding, and one caused by septic shock and attributed to the severity of the patient's underlying liver disease rather than directly to the antiviral treatment.[63] In another series of 23 patients with post-LT severe cholestatic HCV treated with SOF and daclatasvir, SVR12 was achieved in 96%.[64]

PRETRANSPLANT VERSUS POSTTRANSPLANT THERAPY: WHICH IS BETTER?

HCV treatment in the peri-LT setting needs to be individualized. Factors of importance include patient severity of cirrhosis, presence of HCC, donor options, and regional wait times. Treatment approaches are predicted to change continuously over the next few years, as clinicians gain more experience with using currently approved DAA combinations in patients both before LT and after LT and with a large published experience with peri-LT therapies. A suggested framework for considering the timing of treatment in a moderate to high MELD region is shown in **Fig. 5**.

Wait-Listed Patients

In patients listed with HCC or with a living donor available, pre-LT treatment with the goal of preventing HCV recurrence is an option to consider. These patients have a fairly predictable time to LT allowing the initiation of therapy in sufficient time to achieve HCV RNA undetectability for 4 or more weeks. Earlier treatment can be considered in patients with HCC and complications of cirrhosis, for whom treatment may improve liver function and facilitate HCC treatment and/or decrease symptoms related to liver decompensation.

For patients with intermediate MELD scores and no living donor option, the benefits and harms of treatment need to be weighed for each patient. Potential benefits of treatment include reversal of decompensation, reduced risk of death on the waiting list, improved quality of life, and avoidance of LT. Potential harms include lack of response and development of resistance, limited access to future therapies, and reduced MELD scores making LT less accessible. Overall, the lack of long-term data on SVR and reversibility of complications of portal hypertension and liver failure are major impediments to decision making. Pre-LT HCV treatment in this group should be considered on a case-by-case basis and may be best suited for those with lower MELD scores (eg, <20) and/or whose complications from portal hypertension are not refractory (see **Fig. 5**). For those with a high MELD score whose LT is imminent, deferral of HCV treatment until after LT is currently the best option.

Post–Liver Transplant Recipients

In the post-LT setting, patients with severe early recurrence (cholestatic variant) or risk factors for progressive disease should be treated early. As safety and experience with early treatment is acquired, earlier initiation of antiviral therapy is likely. In resource-constrained settings, monitoring of patients with annual liver biopsies or elastography with initiation of treatment if F2 or greater fibrosis is a reasonable strategy. However,

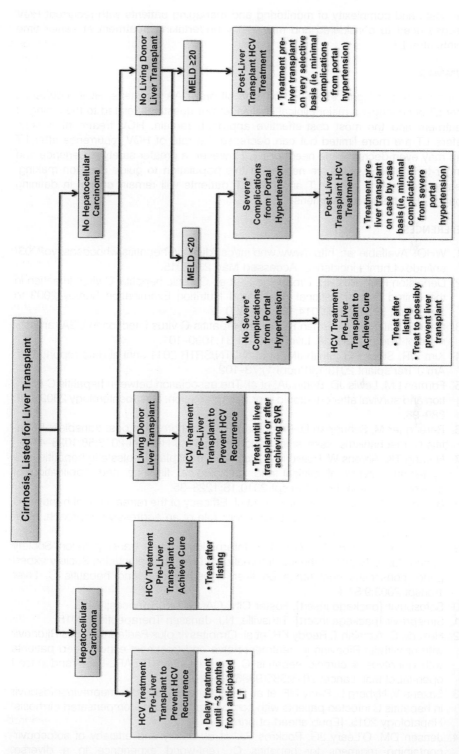

Fig. 5. Suggested approach to HCV treatment in pre-LT patients. [a] Severe complications from portal hypertension are generally medically refractory ascites or encephalopathy.

the costs and complexity of monitoring and managing patients with recurrent HCV disease need to considered and may justify undertaking treatment at earlier time points after LT.

SUMMARY

In the era of the highly effective and safe all-oral DAA regimens, HCV recurrence after LT is no longer a major clinical challenge; but questions related to the timing of treatment and the most cost-effective approach remain. HCV treatment options before LT are more limited but can decrease the rate of HCV recurrence after LT and may even decrease the need for LT. However, a greater safety experience and longer-term efficacy data are needed in this population to guide decision making. Real-world cohorts of pre-LT and post-LT patients will remain critical in defining optimal HCV treatment regimens.

REFERENCES

1. WHO. Available at: http://www.who.int/csr/disease/hepatitis/whocdscsrlyo2003/en/index4.html - incidence. Accessed May 23, 2015.
2. Denniston MM, Jiles RB, Drobeniuc J, et al. Chronic hepatitis C virus infection in the United States, National Health and Nutrition Examination Survey 2003 to 2010. Ann Intern Med 2014;160:293–300.
3. Chak E, Talal AH, Sherman KE, et al. Hepatitis C virus infection in USA: an estimate of true prevalence. Liver Int 2011;31:1090–101.
4. Kim WR, Stock PG, Smith JM, et al. OPTN/SRTR 2011 annual data report: liver. Am J Transplant 2013;13(Suppl 1):73–102.
5. Forman LM, Lewis JD, Berlin JA, et al. The association between hepatitis C infection and survival after orthotopic liver transplantation. Gastroenterology 2002;122:889–96.
6. Berenguer M, Schuppan D. Progression of liver fibrosis in post-transplant hepatitis C: mechanisms, assessment and treatment. J Hepatol 2013;58:1028–41.
7. Narang TK, Ahrens W, Russo MW. Post-liver transplant cholestatic hepatitis C: a systematic review of clinical and pathological findings and application of consensus criteria. Liver Transpl 2010;16:1228–35.
8. Berenguer M, Roche B, Aguilera V, et al. Efficacy of the retreatment of hepatitis C virus infections after liver transplantation: role of an aggressive approach. Liver Transpl 2013;19:69–77.
9. Wiesner RH, Sorrell M, Villamil F, International Liver Transplantation Society Expert Panel. Report of the first International Liver Transplantation Society expert panel consensus conference on liver transplantation and hepatitis C. Liver Transpl 2003;9:S1–9.
10. Sofosbuvir [package insert]. Foster City, CA: Gilead Sciences; 2013.
11. Simeprevir [package insert]. Titusville, NJ: Janssen Therapeutics; 2015.
12. Hezode C, Asselah T, Reddy KR, et al. Ombitasvir plus Paritaprevir plus Ritonavir with or without Ribavirin in treatment-naive and treatment-experienced patients with genotype 4 chronic hepatitis C virus infection (PEARL-I): a randomized open-label trial. Lancet 2015;385(9986):2502–9.
13. Saxena V, Nyberg L, Pauly MP, et al. Safety and efficacy of simeprevir/sofosbuvir in hepatitis C infected patients with compensated and decompensated cirrhosis. Hepatology 2015. [Epub ahead of print].
14. Jensen DM, O'Leary JG, Pockros PJ, et al. Safety and efficacy of sofosbuvir-containing regimens for hepatitis C: real-world experience in a diverse,

longitudinal observational cohort. Program and abstracts of the 65th Annual Meeting of the American Association for the Study of Liver Diseases. Boston (MA), November 7–11, 2014. [abstract: 45].

15. Reddy KR, Lim JK, Kuo A, et al. All oral HCV therapy is safe and effective in patients with decompensated cirrhosis: report from HCV-TARGET. Program and abstracts of the 50th Annual Meeting of the European Association for the Study of the Liver. Vienna (Austria), April 22–26, 2015. [abstract: O005].

16. Stine JG, Intagliata N, Shah NL, et al. Hepatic decompensation likely attributable to simeprevir in patients with advanced cirrhosis. Dig Dis Sci 2015;60: 1031–5.

17. Saxena V, Terrault NA, Hepatitis C. Direct antiviral drugs and hepatic decompensation in patients with advanced cirrhosis: culprit or innocent bystander? Dig Dis Sci 2015;60:806–9.

18. Ledipasvir/sofosbuvir [package insert]. Foster City, CA: Gilead Sciences; 2015.

19. Charlton M, Everson GT, Flamm SL, et al. SOLAR-1 Investigators. Ledipasvir and Sofosbuvir plus Ribavirin for treatment of HCV infection in patients with advanced liver disease. Gastroenterology 2015. [Epub ahead of print].

20. Gane E, Hyland R, An D, et al. Sofosbuvir/ledipasvir fixed dose combination is safe and effective in difficult-to-treat populations including genotype-3 patients, decompensated genotype-1 patients, and genotype-1 patients with prior sofosbuvir treatment experience. Program and abstracts of the 49th Annual Meeting of the European Association for the Study of the Liver. London (United Kingdom), April 9–13, 2014. [abstract: 06].

21. Manns M, Forns X, Samuel D, et al. Ledipasvir/sofosbuvir with ribavirin is safe and efficacious in decompensated and post-liver transplantation patients with HCV infection: preliminary results of the SOLAR-2 trial. Program and abstracts of the 50th Annual Meeting of the European Association for the Study of the Liver. Vienna (Austria), April 22–26, 2015. [abstract: G02].

22. Reddy KR, Bourliere M, Sulkowski MS, et al. Ledipasvir and Sofosbuvir in patients with genotype 1 hepatitis C virus infection and compensated cirrhosis: an integrated safety and efficacy analysis. Hepatology 2015;62(1):79–86.

23. Daclatasvir [package insert]. New York City, NY: Bristol-Myers Squibb; 2014.

24. Hézode C, De Ledinghen V, Fontaine H, et al. Daclatasvir plus sofosbuvir with or without ribavirin in patients with HCV genotype 3 infection: interim analysis of a French multicenter compassionate use program. Program and abstracts of the 50th Annual Meeting of the European Association for the Study of the Liver. Vienna (Austria), April 22–26, 2015. [abstract: LP05].

25. Foster GR, McLauchlan J, Irving W, et al. Treatment of decompensated HCV cirrhosis in patients with diverse genotypes: 12 weeks sofosbuvir and NS5A inhibitors with/without ribavirin is effective in HCV genotypes 1 and 3. Program and abstracts of the 50th Annual Meeting of the European Association for the Study of the Liver. Vienna (Austria), April 22–26, 2015. [abstract: O002].

26. Poordad F, Schiff ER, Vierling JM, et al. Daclatasvir, sofosbuvir, and ribavirin combination for HCV patients with advanced cirrhosis or post-transplant recurrence: ALLY-1 phase 3 study. Program and abstracts of the 50th Annual Meeting of the European Association for the Study of the Liver. Vienna (Austria), April 22–26, 2015. [abstract: L08].

27. D'Ambrosio R, Aghemo A, Rumi MG, et al. A morphometric and immunohistochemical study to assess the benefit of a sustained virological response in hepatitis C virus patients with cirrhosis. Hepatology 2012;56:532–43.

28. Mallet V, Gilgenkrantz H, Serpaggi J, et al. Brief communication: the relationship of regression of cirrhosis to outcome in chronic hepatitis C. Ann Intern Med 2008; 149:399–403.
29. Iacobellis A, Siciliano M, Perri F, et al. Peginterferon alfa-2b and ribavirin in patients with hepatitis C virus and decompensated cirrhosis: a controlled study. J Hepatol 2007;46:206–12.
30. Afdhal N, Everson G, Calleja J, et al. Sofosbuvir and ribavirin for the treatment chronic HCV with cirrhosis and portal hypertension with and without decompensation: early virologic response and safety. Program and abstracts of the 49th Annual Meeting of the European Association for the Study of the Liver. London (United Kingdom), April 9–13, 2014. [abstract: O68].
31. Everson GT. Treatment of patients with hepatitis C virus on the waiting list. Liver Transpl 2003;9:S90–4.
32. Everson GT, Trotter J, Forman L, et al. Treatment of advanced hepatitis C with a low accelerating dosage regimen of antiviral therapy. Hepatology 2005;42: 255–62.
33. Tekin F, Gunsar F, Karasu Z, et al. Safety, tolerability, and efficacy of pegylated-interferon alfa-2a plus ribavirin in HCV-related decompensated cirrhotics. Aliment Pharmacol Ther 2008;27:1081–5.
34. Thomas RM, Brems JJ, Guzman-Hartman G, et al. Infection with chronic hepatitis C virus and liver transplantation: a role for interferon therapy before transplantation. Liver Transpl 2003;9:905–15.
35. Forns X, Garcia-Retortillo M, Serrano T, et al. Antiviral therapy of patients with decompensated cirrhosis to prevent recurrence of hepatitis C after liver transplantation. J Hepatol 2003;39:389–96.
36. Everson GT, Terrault NA, Lok AS, et al. A randomized controlled trial of pretransplant antiviral therapy to prevent recurrence of hepatitis C after liver transplantation. Hepatology 2013;57:1752–62.
37. Carrion JA, Martinez-Bauer E, Crespo G, et al. Antiviral therapy increases the risk of bacterial infections in HCV-infected cirrhotic patients awaiting liver transplantation: a retrospective study. J Hepatol 2009;50:719–28.
38. Massoumi H, Elsiesy H, Khaitova V, et al. An escalating dose regimen of pegylated interferon and ribavirin in HCV cirrhotic patients referred for liver transplant. Transplantation 2009;88:729–35.
39. Hezode C, Fontaine H, Dorival C, et al. Triple therapy in treatment-experienced patients with HCV-cirrhosis in a multicentre cohort of the French Early Access Programme (ANRS CO20-CUPIC) - NCT01514890. J Hepatol 2013;59:434–41.
40. Saxena V, Manos MM, Yee HS, et al. Telaprevir or boceprevir triple therapy in patients with chronic hepatitis C and varying severity of cirrhosis. Aliment Pharmacol Ther 2014;39:1213–24.
41. Jacobson IM, Gordon SC, Kowdley KV, et al. Sofosbuvir for hepatitis C genotype 2 or 3 in patients without treatment options. N Engl J Med 2013;368:1867–77.
42. Osinusi A, Meissner EG, Lee YJ, et al. Sofosbuvir and ribavirin for hepatitis C genotype 1 in patients with unfavorable treatment characteristics: a randomized clinical trial. JAMA 2013;310:804–11.
43. Lawitz E, Mangia A, Wyles D, et al. Sofosbuvir for previously untreated chronic hepatitis C infection. N Engl J Med 2013;368:1878–87.
44. Curry MP, Forns X, Chung RT, et al. Sofosbuvir and ribavirin prevent recurrence of HCV infection after liver transplantation: an open-label study. Gastroenterology 2015;148:100–7.e1.

45. AASLD/IDSA/IAS-USA. Recommendations for testing, managing, and treating hepatitis C. Available at: http://www.hcvguidelines.org. Accessed March 5, 2015.
46. Garcia-Retortillo M, Forns X, Feliu A, et al. Hepatitis C virus kinetics during and immediately after liver transplantation. Hepatology 2002;35:680–7.
47. Terrault N, Shrestha R, Satapathy SK, et al. LP17: Novel approach for the prevention of recurrent hepatitis C in liver transplant recipients: preliminary results from ongoing phase III trial with Civacir®. J Hepatology 2015;62(Suppl 2):S271–2.
48. Berenguer M, Palau A, Aguilera V, et al. Clinical benefits of antiviral therapy in patients with recurrent hepatitis C following liver transplantation. Am J Transplant 2008;8:679–87.
49. Bzowej N, Nelson DR, Terrault NA, et al. PHOENIX: a randomized controlled trial of peginterferon alfa-2a plus ribavirin as a prophylactic treatment after liver transplantation for hepatitis C virus. Liver Transpl 2011;17:528–38.
50. Wang CS, Ko HH, Yoshida EM, et al. Interferon-based combination anti-viral therapy for hepatitis C virus after liver transplantation: a review and quantitative analysis. Am J Transplant 2006;6:1586–99.
51. Burton JR Jr, O'Leary JG, Verna EC, et al. A US multicenter study of hepatitis C treatment of liver transplant recipients with protease-inhibitor triple therapy. J Hepatol 2014;61:508–14.
52. Verna EC, Saxena V, Burton JR Jr, et al, for the CRUSH-C Consortium. Telaprevir- and boceprevir-based triple therapy for hepatitis C in liver transplant recipients with advanced recurrent disease: a multicenter study. Transplantation 2015. [Epub ahead of print].
53. Pungpapong S, Aqel BA, Koning L, et al. Multicenter experience using telaprevir or boceprevir with peginterferon and ribavirin to treat hepatitis C genotype 1 after liver transplantation. Liver Transpl 2013;19:690–700.
54. Charlton M, Gane E, Manns MP, et al. Sofosbuvir and ribavirin for treatment of compensated recurrent hepatitis C virus infection after liver transplantation. Gastroenterology 2015;148:108–17.
55. Tischer S, Fontana RJ. Drug-drug interactions with oral anti-HCV agents and idiosyncratic hepatotoxicity in the liver transplant setting. J Hepatol 2014;60:872–84.
56. Pungpapong S, Aqel B, Leise M, et al. Multicenter experience using sofosbuvir and simeprevir with/without ribavirin to treat hepatitis C genotype 1 after liver transplantation. Hepatology 2015;61(6):1880–6.
57. Brown RS, Reddy K, O'Leary JG, et al. Safety and efficacy of new DAA-based therapy for hepatitis C post-transplant: interval results from the HCV-TARGET longitudinal, observational study. Program and abstracts of the 65th Annual Meeting of the American Association for the Study of Liver Diseases. Boston (MA), November 7–11, 2014. [abstract: LB-4].
58. Janssen R&D (Posted 2013). A study of pharmacokinetics, efficacy, safety, tolerability, of the combination of simeprevir (TMC435), daclatasvir (BMS-790052), and ribavirin (RBV) in patients with recurrent chronic hepatitis C genotype 1b infection after orthotopic liver transplantation (NCT01938625). Available at: http://www.clinicaltrials.gov/ct2/show/NCT01938625. Accessed September 5, 2014.
59. Kwo P, Mantry P, Coakley E, et al. An interferon-free antiviral regimen for HCV after liver transplantation. N Engl J Med 2014;371(25):2375–82.
60. Bifano M, Adamczyk R, Hwang C, et al. Daclatasvir pharmacokinetics in healthy subjects: no clinically-relevant drug-drug interactions with either cyclosporine or tacrolimus. Program and abstracts of the 65th Annual Meeting of the American Association for the Study of Liver Diseases. Boston (MA), November 7–11, 2014. [abstract: 1081].

61. Forns X, Charlton M, Dening J, et al. Sofosbuvir compassionate use program for patients with severe recurrent hepatitis C after liver transplantation. Hepatology 2015;61(5):1485–94.

62. Brown RS, Reddy KR, O'Leary JG, et al. Safety and efficacy of new DAA-based therapy for hepatitis C post-transplant: interval results from the HCV-TARGET longitudinal, observational study. American Association for the Study of Liver Diseases (AASLD) Liver Meeting. Boston (MA), November 7–12, 2014. [abstract: LB-4].

63. Pellicelli AM, Montalbano M, Lionetti R, et al. Sofosbuvir plus daclatasvir for post-transplant recurrent hepatitis C: potent antiviral activity but no clinical benefit if treatment is given late. Dig Liver Dis 2014;46:923–7.

64. Leroy V, Dumortier J, Coilly A, et al. Efficacy of Sofosbuvir and Daclatasvir in patients with fibrosing cholestatic hepatitis C after liver transplantation. Clin Gastroenterol Hepatol 2015. [Epub ahead of print].

Regimens for Patients Coinfected with Human Immunodeficiency Virus

David L. Wyles, MD

KEYWORDS

• HCV • HIV • Treatment • Drug interactions

KEY POINTS

- Accelerated disease progression and the prominent role of hepatitis C virus (HCV)–related liver disease morbidity and mortality in patients with human immunodeficiency virus (HIV) dictate aggressive HCV treatment approaches in this population.
- The efficacy and tolerability of interferon-free direct-acting antiviral (DAA) regimens are equivalent in a coinfected population.
- Drug-drug interactions are a major consideration in deciding on the appropriate HCV DAA regimen in HIV coinfection; some patients require a switch in antiretroviral therapy.
- Additional data are needed in HCV regimens that can be coadministered with HIV protease inhibitors (PIs) boosted with ritonavir.

INTRODUCTION

Hepatitis C virus (HCV) infection in patients with human immunodeficiency virus (HIV) 1, hereafter referred to as HIV coinfection, is significantly more prevalent than in the general population because of shared risk factors for transmission. Global estimates of HCV prevalence in those with HIV range from 15% to 30%, with an estimated 5 million to 7 million persons coinfected with HIV worldwide.[1–4] Patients coinfected with HIV were identified as a special population during the interferon treatment era because of several characteristics, including an accelerated liver disease progression phenotype and inferior responses to HCV treatment with amplified side effect manifestations.[5–11] The arrival of potent interferon-free therapies for HCV has leveled the playing field in terms of antiviral responses to HCV therapy in HIV coinfection. However,

Disclosures: Dr D.L. Wyles has received research grants for the conduct of clinical trials (paid to UC Regents) from AbbVie, Bristol-Myers Squibb, Gilead, Merck, and Tacere. Dr D.L. Wyles has served as a paid consultant to Bristol-Myers Squibb and AbbVie.
Division of Infectious Diseases, UCSD, 9500 Gilman Drive, MC 0711, La Jolla, CA 92093, USA
E-mail address: dwyles@ucsd.edu

other special considerations in this population, including management of drug-drug interactions (DDIs) and maintenance of HIV control, have an expanded importance in the direct-acting antiviral (DAA) era.

Epidemiology and Natural History of Hepatitis C Virus in Patients with Human Immunodeficiency Virus 1

In the past, shared risk factors for both HCV and HIV infection have centered on percutaneous exposures to blood or blood-derived products contaminated with viral RNA. Such exposures include injection drug use and transfusion before widespread screening for HIV and HCV. However, in recent years a unique predilection for sexual transmission of HCV in HIV-positive men who have sex with men was described and is now a recognized, common mode of HCV acquisition in this population.[12,13] These characteristics make discussions of treatment of acute HCV infection and the notion of HCV treatment as prevention of transmission uniquely applicable to a coinfected population.

Compounding the impact of high HCV prevalence in patients with HIV is the accelerated disease course in this population.[6,14] Liver-related disease, most of which is caused by HCV, is a major cause of non–AIDS mortality in those with HIV, second only to non-HIV–related malignancies, accounting for 13% of the deaths seen in a cohort of more than 49,000 persons.[15] Numerous studies have shown an accelerated fibrosis progression rate as well as more frequent decompensation and death once cirrhosis is present.[5,14,16–18] These characteristics highlight the importance of early recognition and treatment of HCV in HIV coinfection. Accordingly, the American Association for the Study of Liver Diseases (AASLD)/Infectious Diseases Society of America (IDSA) HCV guidance document identifies patients with HIV coinfection as a priority population that should be treated for HCV without regard to fibrosis stage.[19]

Special Consideration in Evaluation of Patients Coinfected with Human Immunodeficiency Virus

Much of the pre-HCV treatment evaluation is no different for patients coinfected with HIV compared with patients monoinfected with HCV. Assessment of liver fibrosis stage is imperative to guide both treatment urgency and duration; disease stage is also key to determining the need for additional testing (eg, screening for hepatocellular carcinoma or esophageal varices). In addition, health insurance plans may also require fibrosis staging before a decision on medication coverage is made. Knowledge of a patient's HCV treatment history and response is also critical to deciding on the appropriate DAA therapy but, again, this is no different than for those with HCV alone.

Unique aspects to the pre-HCV treatment evaluation in patients with HIV coinfection are listed in **Table 1**. Given the paramount importance of drug interactions and the likelihood that many patients will require a change in antiretroviral (ARV) therapy to accommodate HCV therapy, a detailed ARV history with special attention to prior HIV virologic failures or results of HIV drug resistance testing are vital. A review of a patient's HIV virologic control can be a useful tool to get an indication of compliance. Intermittent HIV blips represent an opportunity to discuss antiviral medication compliance, for both HIV and HCV. In addition, given the potential interaction and side effect profile of tenofovir disoproxil fumarate (TDF), clinicians should pay special attention to patients' creatinine levels as well as considering a urinalysis to assess for protein or other signs of renal dysfunction.

Table 1	
Special baseline evaluation consideration in patients with HIV coinfection	
Parameter	**Comments**
CD4 cell count	Routine assessment; no indication that CD4 counts affect HCV treatment responses with DAAs
HIV viral load	Review historical trend for an indication of compliance; in general, HIV viral load should be undetectable in patients starting HCV therapy (but not required)
ARV history/resistance	Attention should be paid to ARV regimens on which the patient experienced virologic failure. HIV resistance testing, when available, should be noted
Total and direct bilirubin levels	Particularly important in patients on ATV, which increases indirect bilirubin levels. Direct bilirubin should be monitored, particularly in those with cirrhosis
Creatinine level, urinalysis	TDF may cause renal injury, and interactions with several DAAs may increase TDF levels. Baseline renal function should be evaluated and followed closely on therapy in those on DAA regimens that can increase TDF levels (see text)
Others	Consider baseline testing for HLA-B5701 to determine whether abacavir may be an option in patients on TDF-containing ARV regimens that will be treated with DAA regimens with the potential to further increase TDF levels

Abbreviations: ARV, antiretroviral; ATV, atazanavir; HLA, human leukocyte antigen; TDF, tenofovir disoproxil fumarate.

Treatment of Hepatitis C Virus in Patients with Human Immunodeficiency Virus Using Interferon-containing Regimens

To understand the impact of current DAA therapies it is illustrative to briefly consider the historical limitations of interferon-based therapy in this population. Multiple studies with pegylated interferon (PEG) plus ribavirin showed low response rates, ranging from 14% to 29%, for HCV genotype 1 infection in subjects coinfected with HIV.[7–9] Despite the lower rates of sustained virologic response (SVR) with interferon-based treatment being presumed to be caused by immunosuppression or immune dysregulation in those with HIV, a specific association with HIV disease state (such as CD4 count or HIV viral load [VL]) was not consistently identified.[20,21] Drug interactions were not a prominent consideration, with the only recommendations being to avoid azidothymidine, ddI and D4T because of interactions with ribavirin.[22–25]

The addition of a single DAA to PEG plus ribavirin appears sufficient to attain SVR rates in an HIV coinfected population equivalent to those seen in HCV monoinfection. Starting with telaprevir and boceprevir and culminating with studies of simeprevir (SMV) or sofosbuvir (SOF) combined with PEG and ribavirin SVR rates in subjects coinfected with HIV have been nearly identical to results in monoinfected populations.[26–29] Despite this, tolerability remained an issue, including some reports showing high rates of severe adverse events with first-generation HCV protease inhibitors when used in coinfected patients in a real-world setting.[30] Although SMV-based and SOF-based interferon-containing regimens are better tolerated, the significant medical contraindications, potential for severe side effects, and lower response rates argue for the abandonment of interferon-based HCV therapies in patients with HIV coinfection, just as for those with HCV alone.[19]

Antiretroviral Therapy Considerations and Drug-Drug Interactions

Drug-drug interactions (DDIs) with HIV ARVs represent the most important unique consideration in treating HCV in patients with HIV coinfection (**Fig. 1**). Some general concepts on drug interaction are discussed here, and some ARV regimens that are either problematic or broadly applicable in the context of HCV therapy with all-DAA regimens are highlighted. Specific interactions are discussed separately.

Most subjects infected with HIV being considered for HCV therapy are likely to be on ARVs. Current HIV treatment guidelines recommend HIV therapy regardless of CD4 count[31,32]; in addition, some studies in coinfected subjects suggest that effective HIV treatment may the slow the progression of HCV disease,[33,34] although this finding has not been universal.[35,36]

In general, concerns regarding DDIs surround 2 phenomena: (1) interactions that reduce the concentrations of antiviral medications, exposing the patient to an increased risk of virologic failure and potentially drug resistance for HIV, HCV, or both; and (2) synergistic toxicities or interactions that increase drug levels, increasing the risk of toxicity and resulting in an increase in treatment-related adverse events and/or side effects. The most prevalent DDIs in a coinfected population concern the cytochrome P (CYP) 450 system (particularly the isoenzyme 3A4) or more complex

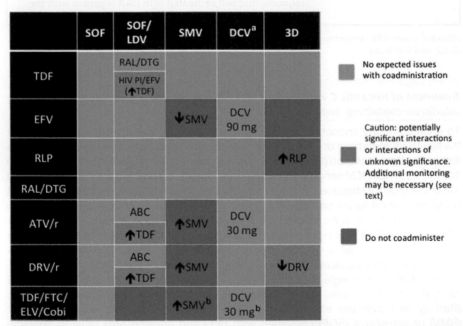

Fig. 1. Interactions between HCV DAAs and common HIV ARVs. Green squares indicate drugs that may be coadministered based on available data or extrapolation; orange squares indicate combinations that may be used if the clinical benefit is thought to outweigh the risk of any potential untoward drug interactions. Combinations in red boxes should generally not be coadministered. Text within boxes indicates drug concentration changes that may be of clinical significance or dose adjustment recommendations. [a]Standard DCV dose is 60mg. [b]Not studied, based on predicted interactions. 3D, 3-DAA regimen (paritaprevir/ritonavir/ombitasvir plus dasabuvir); ATV, atazanavir; Cobi, cobicistat; DCV, daclatasvir; DRV, darunavir; DTG, dolutegravir; EFV, efavirenz; ELV, elvitegravir; FTC, emtricitabine; RAL, raltegravir; RLP, rilpivirine; SOF/LDV, SOF/ledipasvir fixed-dose combination.

multiple drug interactions that may lead to increased levels of TDF and potentially increase the risk of TDF-associated renal injury. Several of the newly recommended first-line HIV regimens contain potent CYP3A4 inhibitors and/or TDF and thus require thorough consideration of DDIs before selecting an HCV treatment regimen[31,32] (see **Fig. 1**). The prominent ARV that is a moderate CYP inducer is Efavirenz (EFV); though no longer a recommended first-line therapy, it remains a commonly used component of ARV regimens. In many cases a switch in ARVs is required to accommodate the optimal HCV regimen for a given patient.

- EFV is a moderate CYP3A4 inducer with the potential to significantly reduce exposure to susceptible coadministered DAAs.
- Ritonavir (RTV or /r when used for boosting) is a potent CYP3A4 inhibitor with the potential to increase exposure to coadministered DAAs.
- As a general rule, nonboosted HIV integrase strand transfer inhibitor (INSTI)–based regimens (composed of an INSTI plus 2 nucleoside reverse transciptase inhibitors [NRTIs]) are conducive to the use of any currently available HCV DAA regimen (see **Fig. 1**).

Moving beyond first-line therapies in treatment-experienced patients infected with HIV, many of whom have extensive ARV exposure histories and drug resistance, the management of DDIs and ability to switch ARV regimens to accommodate HCV DAA treatment is complex and not amenable to an algorithmic approach in deciding on ARV-DAA therapy combinations. In general, these patients should be managed in a team setting in conjunction with an experienced HIV clinician and a clinical pharmacist.

Current Regimens for Hepatitis C Virus Genotype 1 Treatment in Patients with Human Immunodeficiency Virus 1

Approved regimens for the treatment of HCV genotype 1 can be broadly categorized as nucleotide based or protease inhibitor based. Data in HIV coinfection are limited in scope with most regimens (**Table 2**), although, as alluded to previously, efficacy and tolerability data in an HCV monoinfected population should be considered widely applicable to patients with HIV coinfection (accounting for the same HCV treatment history and fibrosis stage). Knowledge of clinically significant DDIs is key to determining the utility and safety of a given regimen for individual patients.

Nucleotide-based Hepatitis C Virus Treatment Regimens

SOF is the only currently approved HCV NS5B nucleotide inhibitor.[37] Studies of SOF in patients with HIV include (1) a pilot study in combination with PEG and ribavirin (RBV),[29] (2) SOF/RBV therapy for genotypes 1 to 4,[38,39] and (3) 2 phase 3 studies of SOF plus non-structural protein 5A (NS5A) inhibitors (ledipasvir [LDV] in ION-4 [NCT02073656] and daclatasvir (DCV) in ALLY-2 [NCT02032888]). The efficacy of SOF-based regimens in HCV monoinfection is discussed by Ayoub and Tran elsewhere in this issue.

Sofosbuvir plus interferon

Twenty-three treatment-naive, noncirrhotic patients coinfected with HIV were treated with SOF plus PEG alfa-2a and weight-based RBV for 12 weeks.[29] Sustained virologic response at 12 (SVR12) and 24 weeks (SVR24) after therapy was achieved in 91% of subjects (21 of 23) with only 1 virologic failure. Most subjects were HCV genotype 1 and the SVR12/SVR24 in this population was 89% (17 of 19). Treatment was well tolerated but 70% of subjects treated experienced an adverse event, including 2 treatment

Table 2
HCV DAA regimens and SVR rates in patients with HIV coinfection

		HCV Regimens Recommended for Use in HIV Coinfection[a]				
		Data in HIV (SVR12, Where Available)				No Data in HIV
Geno-type		SOF/RBV	SOF/LDV	3D + RBV[d]	SOF/DCV[b]	SOF/SMV
1	Naive, NC	Not recommended	12 wk TN (C + NC): 95% (n = 146)	12 wk	97% (n = 72)	12 wk
	Naive, C	TN = 81% Cirrhosis = 64%	12 wk	12/24 wk (1b/1a)	89% (n = 9)	24 wk
	Exp, NC		12 wk	12 wk	100% (n = 28)	12 wk
	Exp, C		TE (C + NC): 97% (n = 181) 24 wk	12/24 wk (1b/1a) 94%[c] (12 wk, n = 31) 91%[c] (24 wk, n = 32)	92% (n = 13)	24 wk
2	—	12 wk TN = 89% TE = 90% (24 wk)	NA	NA	100% (n = 13)	NA
3	—	24 wk TN = 67% (12 wk) TN = 91% (24 wk) TE = 88% (24 wk)	NA	NA	100% (n = 10)	NA

Abbreviations: 3D, 3 DAA regimen; C, cirrhosis; DCV, daclatasvir; Exp, experienced; LDV, ledipasvir; NA, not available; NC, noncirrhotic; SMV, simeprevir; TE, treatment experienced; TN, treatment naive.

a See **Fig. 1** for limitations.
b Only available in the European Union.
c Mixed population of treatment naive, treatment experienced, cirrhotic, and noncirrhotic.
d Only studied with RBV thus far in HIV. RBV not likely to be needed in genotype 1b.

discontinuations caused by adverse event (mood disturbance and anemia). This finding is consistent with the known poor tolerability and side effect profile of PEG plus RBV. These efficacy and tolerability results are comparable with the phase 3 NEUTRINO study[40]; however, given the available alternatives with better tolerability and numerically higher SVR rates, this regimen is not recommended for treatment of HCV genotype 1 in patients with HIV in most settings.[19]

Sofosbuvir plus RBV

Two phase 3 studies evaluated the safety and efficacy of SOF plus weight-based RBV in HIV coinfection for treatment of HCV genotypes 1 to 4.[38,39] In PHOTON 1, treatment-naive genotype 1 subjects and treatment-experienced genotype 2 and genotype 3 subjects were treated for 24 weeks with SOF plus RBV.[38] Naive genotype 2/genotype 3 subjects were treated with the same regimen for 12 weeks. Many ARV regimens were allowed provided the NRTIs were tenofovir/emtricitabine (FTC).

PHOTON 2 used a similar treatment approach with the notable exceptions that genotype 4 was included (treated for 24 weeks) and that treatment-naive genotype 3 subjects were treated for 24 weeks, consistent with the current label for SOF.[39] Genotype 2 treatment-experienced patients were treated for 24 weeks in both PHOTON studies, in contrast with the current label indication for SOF/RBV in patients with genotype 2.[37] Again, most HIV ARVs were allowed; TDF and FTC or lamivudine (3TC) were the only nucleosides/nucleotides allowed. Other HIV characteristics for inclusion included a CD4 count greater than 200 cells/mm³ with a suppressed HIV viral load (<50 copies/mL) or CD4 count greater than 500 cells/mm³ for subjects not on ARV therapy (ART). Compensated cirrhosis was allowed in both studies with about 20% of subjects in each study being cirrhotic, although only approximately 10% of patients with genotype 1 were cirrhotic. A summary of the SVR12 rates from the 2 PHOTON studies includes:

- Genotype 1: 81% (182 of 226) with 17% relapse rate
- Genotype 2 (naive/experienced): 89% (40 of 45)/90% (27 of 30) with a 2%/7% relapse rate
- Genotype 3 (naive, 12 weeks): 67% (28 of 42) with a 29% relapse rate
- Genotype 3 (naive/experienced, 24 weeks): 91% (52 of 57)/88% (58 of 66) with a 7%/11% relapse rate
- Genotype 4: 84% (26 of 31) with a 16% relapse rate

As expected, response rates were lower in patients with cirrhosis; in particular, genotype 3 treatment-experienced cirrhotics had an SVR12 rate of 79%. The regimen was well tolerated with the expected anemia related to RBV and increased rates of hyperbilirubinemia in patients on atazanavir (ATV). HIV control was maintained, with the only confirmed HIV viral breakthroughs (n = 2) occurring in patients with documented noncompliance with their HIV therapy.

Although the genotype 1 response rates in the PHOTON studies were as expected, the availability of more efficacious therapies dictate that, in general, this regimen should not be used for subjects coinfected with genotype 1 and HIV.[19] The exception may be the rare HIV treatment-experienced patients on ART regimens that cannot be modified to accommodate a more potent DAA regimen without significant risk of losing HIV control. However, even in this setting, a more potent HCV DAA regimen with potentially significant drug interactions may be chosen, particularly in patients who are difficult to treat or who have advanced fibrosis. In this setting, consultation with an HCV treatment expert is prudent, with treatment approaches determined on a case-by-case basis.

In the combined PHOTON studies, SVR rates for genotypes 2 and 3 were comparable with those seen in FISSION, FUSION, POSITRON, and VALENCE, and treatment recommendations for these genotypes are the same as for patients monoinfected with HCV.[19,37,40-42] The PHOTON results also further support that a 24 week duration is optimal should a SOF/RBV regimen be chosen for genotype 3 infection. As indicated in recent guidance updates, the addition of DCV or PEG to SOF/RBV may be optimal for many genotype 3 infected patients.[19]

Sofosbuvir-antiretroviral drug interactions
SOF has a limited drug interaction potential because it is not a substrate or inhibitor of the CYP system, making it an attractive component of regimens to use in HIV coinfection.[37,43] SOF is a substrate of the P-glycoprotein (P-gp) drug export pump and thus there is potential for decreased SOF exposure when coadministered with potent P-gp inducers.

- Tipranavir is a potent P-gp inducer and SOF should not be coadministered with this infrequently used HIV PI.[37]

The favorable DDI profile of SOF in combination with various ARVs was shown in an interaction study that enrolled 38 subjects coinfected with HIV/HCV.[29] Notably, no significant interaction for any of the ARVs studied (EFV, FTC, tenofovir, zidovudine, lamivudine, ATV, RTV, darunavir (DRV), or raltegravir [RAL]) were found. Note that TDF exposure was increased when coadministered with SOF. The increase in TDF exposure was modest (20%–30% increase in area under the concentration-time curve [AUC]) and unlikely to be of clinical significance in itself. However, this interaction must be kept in mind when SOF and TDF are coadministered in the setting of other agents that also increase TDF; here the cumulative effect may have clinical relevance.

Sofosbuvir plus an NS5A inhibitor
SOF coformulated with LDV is US Food and Drug Administration approved for treatment of HCV genotype 1 infection.[44] Recently, the first results from a phase III study of SOF/LDV (400 mg/90 mg) given for 12 weeks without RBV in patients coinfected with HIV were published.[45] The single-arm ION-4 study enrolled 335 treatment-naive or treatment-experienced coinfected subjects with genotype 1 (n = 327) or 4 (n = 8) HCV infection. Subjects were required to be on one of 3 allowable ART regimens: TDF/FTC with either RAL, RLP, or EFV. Other entry criteria included a CD4 count of greater than 100 cells/mm^3, HIV viral load less than 50 copies/mL, and a creatinine clearance (CrCl) of greater than 60 mL/min; patients with compensated cirrhosis were allowed to enroll.

Demographic features of the population studied include 34% African American, 55% treatment experienced, and 20% with cirrhosis. Overall excellent efficacy and tolerability/safety results were seen:

- SVR12 was achieved by 96% in genotype 1 (96% overall, including genotypes 1 and 4).
  - SVR12 by 95%/97% in treatment naive and experienced, respectively
  - SVR12 by 96%/94% in noncirrhotic and cirrhotic patients, respectively
- No treatment discontinuations caused by adverse events.
  - No confirmed HIV virologic failures

A pilot study (NIH ERADICATE study) reported similar results in 49 subjects coinfected with HIV with genotype 1 HCV treated for 12 weeks with SOF/LDV (400/90 mg).[46] All subjects were treatment naive and those with cirrhosis were excluded.

As in ION-4, ARV regimens included TDF/FTC with EFV, RLP, or RAL; 13 of 49 subjects were not on ART.

- SVR12 by 98% of subjects with only 1 virologic relapse.
- Responses were similar in treated and untreated subjects with HIV and therapy was well tolerated.

The only patient to experience HIV viral load breakthrough had documented noncompliance with ARVs.

DCV, a potent pangenotypic NS5A inhibitor, is an attractive option for use in HIV coinfection because of a well-defined DDI profile and preliminary dosing approaches for many ARV regimens.[47,48] DCV was recently approved in the United States; DCV has been available in the European Union with guidelines for its use in patients with HIV coinfection.[49]

Efficacy data from a phase III trial (ALLY-2, NCT02032888) in coinfected patients show excellent response rates in this population in line with other HCV monoinfected and coinfected data for SOF plus an NS5A inhibitor.[45,50–52] In the ALLY-2 study coinfected treatment-naive patients, including patients with cirrhosis, were randomized 2:1 to treatment with SOF 400 mg plus DCV (30, 60, or 90 mg depending on concomitant ARVs) for 12 (n = 101) or 8 weeks (n = 50).[53] A third arm enrolling treatment-experienced patients (n = 52) only evaluated 12 weeks of therapy. All HCV genotypes were allowed (although only genotypes 1–4 were enrolled) and patients on most ART regimens were eligible except those on a mixed CYP inducer/inhibitor–based regimen (eg, EFV combined with a ritonavir-boosted PI). DCV was dosed at 30 mg in all subjects on ritonavir-boosted HIV PIs (discussed later), 90 mg in patients on EFV or nevirapine, and 60 mg for all others. Patients were required to have a CD4 count greater than 100 cells/mm^3 with HIV viral load less than 50 copies/mL, as well as CrCl greater than 50 mL/min.

Key demographic features of the overall population included 34% African American and 14% with cirrhosis, including 29% with cirrhosis in the treatment-experienced arm. Again, excellent results were seen:

- SVR12 by 97% of patients with genotype 1 treated for 12 weeks
  - SVR12 by 96%/98% in treatment naive and experienced, respectively
  - SVR12 by 98%/91% in noncirrhotic and cirrhotic patients, respectively
- All patients with other than genotype 1 achieved SVR12 in the 12-week arms
  - Genotype 2 (n = 13), genotype 3 (n = 10, and genotype 4 (n = 3)
- SVR12 by 76% of patients with genotype 1 treated for 8 weeks
  - The same 76% SVR12 was found when including all genotypes treated for 8 weeks
- No treatment discontinuations caused by adverse events
  - Two patients with HIV VL greater than 400 copies/mL
    - One patient incarcerated and lost to follow-up
    - One patient resuppressed with resumption of the same ART regimen

This study was the first to examine a shorter, 8-week treatment duration and raises some potential concerns with truncating treatment duration in patients with HIV coinfection. The inclusion of cirrhotic patients in the 8-week arm as well as the potential for lower DCV exposure in patients on DRV or lopinavir (LPV) may partially account for the lower SVR12 rate; however, it is possible that HIV coinfection may adversely affect HCV treatment responses as the lower limit of treatment duration is explored. Pending additional data, it seems premature to routinely treat patients coinfected with HIV otherwise meeting criteria (treatment naive, noncirrhotic with HCV RNA <6 million IU/mL) for truncated therapy with 8 weeks of SOF plus an NS5A inhibitor.

NS5A inhibitor drug interactions and implications for sofosbuvir/NS5A regimens
Despite the same antiviral mechanism of action, LDV and DCV interact with common metabolic pathways and transporters differently and thus have a different potential for significant DDI when combined with ARVs.[48,54] LDV does not undergo metabolism via, or inhibit, the CYP450 system. Systemic exposure is primarily to unchanged drug with elimination in the feces. LDV does inhibit transporters, including P-gp and BCRP (breast cancer resistance protein), and may increase levels of coadministered drugs that are also substrates for these transporters. It is also a substrate for P-gp. Despite this fairly benign metabolic profile, changes in TDF exposure were seen during SOF/ LDV coadministration with TDF/FTC/RLP, and in particular with TDF/FTC/EFV.[44,54] TDF exposure (administered as TDF/FTC/EFV) was increased by 98% when coadministered with SOF/LDV. This change is greater than that seen with SOF alone or when TDF is combined with ritonavir-boosted HIV PIs.[43,55] The clinical significance is unclear but monitoring of renal function during coadministration is required.

Although the mechanism is unclear, coadministration of LDV (as SOF/LDV) with DRV/r or ATV/r results in a 34% and 113% increase in LDV AUC, respectively, and a 45% and 98% increase in C_{max} (maximum concentration), respectively.[44,54] LDV has a high therapeutic index and thus increases in exposure to this degree are not anticipated to have untoward clinical effects. Importantly, what is currently unknown is how more complex multiple drug interactions in clinical practice may affect drug levels, particularly of TDF, and safety/adverse effects encountered during treatment with SOF/LDV. Drug interaction studies with SOF/LDV and ritonavir-boosted HIV PI regimens also containing TDF are underway; thus far, these patients have been excluded from all clinical studies of SOF/LDV in HIV coinfection. Concern about this interaction is reflected in the label for SOF/LDV, where it is recommended that alternative therapies be considered in patients on ritonavir-boosted HIV PIs.[44] In select patients, because of advanced HCV-related liver disease or a lack of alternative HIV therapies, coadministration of SOF/LDV with HIV PIs and TDF may be advisable, provided that close monitoring for TDF-related toxicity is undertaken. However, this approach is potentially risky in patients with underlying renal dysfunction or factors predisposing them to renal injury, such as hypertension or diabetes mellitus. In addition, in patients requiring HIV PIs who are going to be treated with SOF/LDV, exchanging abacavir (ABC) for TDF can be considered in appropriate patients (eg, human leukocyte antigen [HLA]–B5701 negative with anticipated or known virus sensitivity to ABC).

In contrast, LDV exposure is reduced by coadministration with EFV (36% decrease in LDV AUC), potentially caused by induction of P-gp or other transporters by EFV.[44,54,56] However, this interaction does not appear to have clinical significance. In the ION-4 study SVR rates were comparable between patients on EFV-based ART (94% SVR) and those on non-EFV-based ART (97% SVR). In addition LDV exposure was no different between patients on EFV and those not on EFV.[45] As with ritonavir-boosted HIV PIs, the increase in TDF exposure seen with LDV and EFV individually requires caution in coadministration to any patients with underlying renal dysfunction or predisposing conditions, and careful monitoring of renal function is recommended.

DCV drug interactions with HIV ARVs have been adequately characterized and offer more flexibility in combining SOF/DCV with multiple HIV regimens.[48,49,57] DCV is metabolized via CYP3A4 and is a P-gp substrate so it is a victim of DDIs but does not seem to be a significant perpetrator of interaction effects, although it is a P-gp, OAT1B1/B3, and BRCP inhibitor. In contrast with LDV, DCV had no impact on TDF exposure during coadministration. EFV, a potent CYP 3A4 inducer, decreases DCV exposure by 32%. ATV/rit coadministration results in a significant increase in DCV exposure (110% increase in AUC), while other ritonavir-boosted PIs (DRV and LPV) do not significantly increase DCV exposure (≤40% increase in AUC).[49,57] Although not studied, the investigators predict that cobicistat would result in a similar increase in DCV exposure and recommend dose adjustment.[57] Combining the available data with extrapolations for ARVs not studied has allowed comprehensive recommendations for DCV dosing in combination with various ARV regimens[57] (see **Fig. 1**).

- Full-dose DCV (60 mg) when combined with LPV or DRV boosted with ritonavir
- DCV (30 mg) recommended with cobicistat-boosted elvitegravir and ritonavir-boosted ATV
- DCV (90 mg) recommended with EFV or nevirapine

Sofosbuvir plus an NS3 protease inhibitor
SMV is approved for use in combination with SOF in an interferon-free combination for treatment of HCV genotype 1 infection.[58] Despite this approval, no clinical trial data are available on this combination in HIV coinfection. Given the availability of this combination in the US since late 2013, it is a certainty that patients coinfected with HIV have been treated with this combination in clinical practice. SMV was well tolerated and efficacious in a phase 3 study of SMV plus PEG/RBV in coinfected patients[28] and clinicians should have no reservations related to the efficacy of SOF/SMV in coinfected patients beyond the knowledge gaps for HCV monoinfection treatment,[59] including:

- Uncertainty over the impact of the Q80K variant
- The role of RBV in this regimen
- The optimal duration of therapy in difficult-to-treat populations such as null responders and patients with cirrhosis.

The major limitation for this regimen unique to patients with HIV is the significant drug interactions between SMV and many common ARV regimens.[60]

SMV is a CYP3A4 substrate and thus inducers and inhibitors of this isoenzyme significantly alter its exposure. SMV is also a moderate inhibitor of intestinal, but not hepatic, CYP3A4, meaning that it may also affect the levels of coadministered drugs, although generally to a lesser extent.[58] Drug interaction studies showed significant decreases in SMV exposure with coadministration with EFV (70% decrease in AUC).[60] In contrast, potent CYP3A4 inhibitors such as ritonavir resulted in more than a 2.5-fold increase in SMV exposure. As a result, SMV should not be coadministered with potent CYP3A4 inducers or inhibitors. Among ARVs this includes inducers such as EFV, nevirapine (and probably etravirine), and inhibitors such as all ritonavir-boosted or cobicistat-boosted HIV ARVs. No significant interactions between SMV and RAL or RLP were found and SMV can be coadministered with RLP or INSTI-based regimens (excluding cobicistat-elvitegravir). In addition, SMV had no impact on TDF exposure (<20% increase in AUC).[60]

NS3 protease inhibitor–based regimens
The 3-DAA regimen (3D) composed of the protease inhibitor paritaprevir boosted with ritonavir (100 mg) in a fixed-dose combination with the NS5A inhibitor ombitasvir plus the NS5B nonnucleoside inhibitor dasabuvir with or without RBV is an efficacious regimen approved for the treatment of HCV genotype 1 infection.[61] Preliminary SVR24 data are available from a phase 2b study of this combination in subjects infected with HIV on ATV or RAL-based ART regimens.[62] TURQUOISE 1 evaluated 3D plus RBV in 63 treatment-naive and treatment-experienced subjects with HCV

genotype 1 coinfected with HIV, including patients with compensated cirrhosis. Subjects were allocated 1:1 to receive 12 (n = 31) or 24 weeks (n = 32) of treatment. SVR12 rates were 94% and 91% for the 12-week and 24-week arms respectively by an ITT (intention to treat) analysis. Importantly, only 2 subjects had documented HCV virologic failure, 1 in each arm, whereas 2 subjects experienced confirmed reinfection and 1 withdrew consent. The regimen was well tolerated with no serious adverse events or discontinuations caused by adverse events. Benign hyperbilirubinemia (primarily indirect) was more frequent in subjects on ATV-containing HIV therapy. Based on these data and extrapolation from HCV monoinfection studies, the same treatment approaches should be used for this regimen in HIV coinfection (see **Table 2**).[61]

The 3D regimen has significant potential for DDIs with ARVs because of the use of ritonavir in the regimen as well as the metabolic profiles of the HCV antivirals themselves.[61] Paritaprevir is a CYP3A4 substrate and thus susceptible to boosting by ritonavir. Dasabuvir is a CYP2C8 substrate. Ombitasvir is not a primary CYP substrate, with limited potential for drug interactions. All component of the regimen are P-gp substrates and should not be coadministered with potent P-gp inducers. Extensive DDI studies have been conducted in healthy volunteers with the 3D regimen and many HIV ARVs.[63,64] A summary of the findings includes (see also **Fig. 1**):

- The non-nucleoside reverse transcriptase inhibitors (NNRTIs) EFV and RLP should not be coadministered with the 3D regimen.
- ATV (and likely DRV) can be safely coadministered with the 3D regimen.
- RAL (and likely dolutegravir [DTG]) can be safely coadministered with the 3D regimen.

Rapid liver function test increases and gastrointestinal intolerance were seen with coadministration of EFV (administered as TDF/FTC/EFV). Rilpivirine trough levels and AUC were increased from 150% to 270% when coadministered with the 3D regimen. Early RLP HIV clinical trials with 75 mg showed similar exposure levels and the potential for significant QTc prolongation (>10 milliseconds), increasing the risk for arrhythmias or cardiac arrest.[65]

All 3D components are inhibitors of UGT1A1 and thus have the potential to increase exposure of RAL and DTG (as well as elvitegravir in the presence of CYP3A4 inhibitors). RAL exposure was increased by 100% to 134% during 3D coadministration.[63] However, because of the high therapeutic index of RAL, no dose adjustment is necessary and the 3D regimen can be given to patients on RAL-based ART. Although no data are currently available, the 3D regimen can likely be safely used in patients on DTG-based regimens as well.

Minimal changes in ATV AUC and trough concentrations (<10%) are seen when it is coadministered with the 3D regimen.[64] Importantly, ATV should be given at 300 mg without the usual ritonavir boosting dose because this is supplied by the 3D regimen. This approach was successfully undertaken in the TURQUOISE-1 coinfection study; however, it is imperative that patients are reminded to resume their ritonavir boosting dose once HCV treatment is completed.

DRV administered as 800 mg in the morning or 600 mg twice a day with an additional 100 mg of ritonavir in the evening plus the 3D regimen resulted in an approximately 20% decrease in DRV AUC and 45% decrease in DRV trough concentrations for both dosing regimens.[64] This change in DRV exposure is unlikely to be clinically significant because concentrations of DRV are considerably greater than the estimated 90% effective concentration (EC90) for most patients with sensitive HIV.[66] However, in patients already on 600 mg twice a day because of HIV resistance, this exposure change can theoretically increase the risk of loss of HIV virologic control.

Until ongoing studies of the 3D regimen in patients on DRV are completed, DRV should not be routinely coadministered with the 3D regimen.[61]

Human Immunodeficiency Virus Control During Direct-acting Antiviral Therapy

Based on the limited clinical trial data available, loss of HIV-1 virologic control has not been an issue with any of the HCV DAA regimens currently available.[46,62] However, extrapolation from clinical trials in carefully selected patients with close monitoring to clinical practice is perilous and clinicians must remain vigilant, particularly if changing HIV regimens to accommodate HCV therapy in a patient with exposure to multiple prior ARVs and/or known HIV drug resistance. Given the nature of the most prevalent DDIs with HCV medications, in many cases this means replacing a boosted PI-based regimen with an HIV regimen that has a lower barrier to resistance and is less forgiving of noncompliance. Necessary historical data and key factors to consider include:

- What is the patient's ARVs exposure history?
- Is there evidence of noncompliance?
- Has the patient experienced HIV virologic failure in the past (or been treated for HIV before the highly active ARV therapy era)?
- Are HIV resistance testing results available and/or is the patient likely to have HIV resistance (eg, failure with a 3TC-containing regimen; likely M184V)?

As shown in the SWITCHMRK studies, patients suppressed on an HIV PI-based regimen who have a history of virologic failure or treatment with more than 1 prior HIV regimen are at an increased risk to experience HIV virologic failure when transitioned to an RAL-based ARV regimen.[67] Whether these considerations also apply to DTG, an INSTI with a higher barrier to resistance and proven efficacy in HIV treatment–experienced patients, is unknown in the context of switching ARVs to accommodate HCV therapy.[68–70]

Strategies that can be considered to accommodate DAA therapy in treatment-experienced patients with HIV currently suppressed on HIV PIs include using high-dose DTG (50 mg twice a day) and/or combining an INSTI with an RLP-based HIV regimen in persons without resistance to NNRTIs. However, it must be emphasized that these strategies have not been evaluated in clinical trials and consultation with an expert in HIV therapy and resistance is recommended before changing regimens in HIV-experienced patients with limited ARV options. The recent availability of an HIV archived resistance test (HIV GenoSure Archive, LabCorp) based on sequencing of integrated proviral DNA is an intriguing option to assist in selecting alternative regimens in patients with long-term HIV suppression but significant prior ARV exposure.[71] Again, the caveat is that there are no clinical trial data using this approach to guide decision making.

SUMMARY

Are patients with HIV coinfection still a special population? Highly efficacious and well-tolerated HCV DAA therapies have revolutionized the treatment of HCV, including its treatment in patients with HIV coinfection. Concerns over inferior treatment responses in patients with HIV no longer exist and regimens proven efficacious in HCV monoinfection are widely applicable to patients with HIV. Thus, from a treatment efficacy standpoint, patients infected with HIV are no longer a special population.

However, several unique considerations remain in this population. First and foremost, drug interactions add a layer of complexity to treating patients with HIV; they are the single most important consideration in formulating an HCV treatment plan in patients on ARVs now that clinicians have several highly effective and well-tolerated DAA options for treating genotype 1 HCV. Additional options and data are needed on the use of DAA regimens in patients on ritonavir-boosted HIV PIs.

Efficacy of current DAA regimens starts to decrease in very difficult-to-treat mono-infected populations (such as prior interferon null responders who also have cirrhosis) or as treatment durations are shortened to less than 12 weeks. Given the increased rate of HCV disease progression and poor response to interferon-based therapies, more data are needed on the effectiveness of DAA therapies at the extremes in patients coinfected with HIV. Whether HCV treatment efficacy will remain similar for patients with HIV who are most difficult to treat or as the lower limits of HCV therapy duration are tested remains unknown.

In addition, as it is for many patients with HCV, access to new therapies is also an issue in patients with HIV. In this scenario, could patients with coinfection have the upper hand? Support services are generally more available and accessible to patients with HIV infection. In addition, in some states, AIDS drug assistance programs cover medication costs for DAAs in patients without other funding sources.

After some initial concerns and suggestions that some health plans may try to prevent HIV providers from prescribing newer HCV medications, this ill-advised approach seems to have largely been abandoned.[72–74] In most respects, HIV providers are well suited to treat HCV in patients with HIV because: (1) they possess knowledge of the use of antiviral medications and management of drug interactions, (2) they are in the best position to make decisions on alterations of ARV therapy if needed, and (3) they are able to provide treatment to patients in a primary care setting. As with any complex disease, a collaborative effort will be required for patients with advanced liver disease or complex drug interaction, incorporating a team approach consisting of HIV specialists, hepatologists, and clinical pharmacists.

The future of HCV treatment looks bright, including for patients with HIV.

REFERENCES

1. Sherman KE, Rouster SD, Chung RT, et al. Hepatitis C virus prevalence among patients infected with human immunodeficiency virus: a cross-sectional analysis of the US adult AIDS Clinical Trials Group. Clin Infect Dis 2002;34(6):831–7.
2. Alter MJ. Epidemiology of viral hepatitis and HIV co-infection. J Hepatol 2006; 44(1 Suppl):S6–9.
3. Soriano V, Vispo E, Labarga P, et al. Viral hepatitis and HIV co-infection. Antiviral Res 2010;85(1):303–15.
4. Puoti M, Moioli M, Travi G, et al. The burden of liver disease in human immunodeficiency virus-infected patients. Semin Liver Dis 2012;32(2):103–13.
5. Benhamou Y, Bochet M, Di Martino V, et al. Liver fibrosis progression in human immunodeficiency virus and hepatitis C virus coinfected patients. The Multivirc Group. Hepatology 1999;30(4):1054–8.
6. Kirk GD, Mehta SH, Astemborski J, et al. HIV, age, and the severity of hepatitis C virus-related liver disease: a cohort study. Ann Intern Med 2013;158(9):658–66.
7. Torriani FJ, Rodriguez-Torres M, Rockstroh JK, et al. Peginterferon alfa-2a plus ribavirin for chronic hepatitis C virus infection in HIV-infected patients. N Engl J Med 2004;351(5):438–50.
8. Chung RT, Andersen J, Volberding P, et al. Peginterferon alfa-2a plus ribavirin versus interferon alfa-2a plus ribavirin for chronic hepatitis C in HIV-coinfected persons. N Engl J Med 2004;351(5):451–9.

9. Carrat F, Bani-Sadr F, Pol S, et al. Pegylated interferon alfa-2b vs standard interferon alfa-2b, plus ribavirin, for chronic hepatitis C in HIV-infected patients: a randomized controlled trial. JAMA 2004;292(23):2839–48.

10. Bani-Sadr F, Lapidus N, Melchior J-C, et al. Severe weight loss in HIV/HCV-coinfected patients treated with interferon plus ribavirin: incidence and risk factors. J Viral Hepat 2008;15(4):255–60.

11. Bani-Sadr F, Carrat F, Rosenthal E, et al. Spontaneous hepatic decompensation in patients coinfected with HIV and hepatitis C virus during interferon-ribavirin combination treatment. Clin Infect Dis 2005;41(12):1806–9.

12. Danta M, Brown D, Bhagani S, et al. Recent epidemic of acute hepatitis C virus in HIV-positive men who have sex with men linked to high-risk sexual behaviours. AIDS Lond Engl 2007;21(8):983–91.

13. Van de Laar TJW, Matthews GV, Prins M, et al. Acute hepatitis C in HIV-infected men who have sex with men: an emerging sexually transmitted infection. AIDS Lond Engl 2010;24(12):1799–812.

14. Graham CS, Baden LR, Yu E, et al. Influence of human immunodeficiency virus infection on the course of hepatitis C virus infection: a meta-analysis. Clin Infect Dis 2001;33(4):562–9.

15. Smith CJ, Ryom L, Weber R, et al. Trends in underlying causes of death in people with HIV from 1999 to 2011 (D: A:D): a multicohort collaboration. Lancet 2014; 384(9939):241–8.

16. Pineda JA, Romero-Gómez M, Díaz-García F, et al. HIV coinfection shortens the survival of patients with hepatitis C virus-related decompensated cirrhosis. Hepatology 2005;41(4):779–89.

17. Pineda JA, Aguilar-Guisado M, Rivero A, et al. Natural history of compensated hepatitis C virus-related cirrhosis in HIV-infected patients. Clin Infect Dis 2009; 49(8):1274–82.

18. López-Diéguez M, Montes ML, Pascual-Pareja JF, et al. The natural history of liver cirrhosis in HIV-hepatitis C virus-coinfected patients. AIDS Lond Engl 2011;25(7): 899–904.

19. Initial treatment of HCV infection [Internet]. Available at: http://www.hcv guidelines.org/full-report/initial-treatment-hcv-infection. Accessed January 4, 2015.

20. Dore GJ, Torriani FJ, Rodriguez-Torres M, et al. Baseline factors prognostic of sustained virological response in patients with HIV-hepatitis C virus co-infection. AIDS Lond Engl 2007;21(12):1555–9.

21. Opravil M, Sasadeusz J, Cooper DA, et al. Effect of baseline CD4 cell count on the efficacy and safety of peginterferon Alfa-2a (40KD) plus ribavirin in patients with HIV/hepatitis C virus coinfection. J Acquir Immune Defic Syndr 1999;47(1): 36–49.

22. Lafeuillade A, Hittinger G, Chadapaud S. Increased mitochondrial toxicity with ribavirin in HIV/HCV coinfection. Lancet 2001;357(9252):280–1.

23. Laguno M, Milinkovic A, de Lazzari E, et al. Incidence and risk factors for mitochondrial toxicity in treated HIV/HCV-coinfected patients. Antivir Ther 2005; 10(3):423–9.

24. Bani-Sadr F, Carrat F, Pol S, et al. Risk factors for symptomatic mitochondrial toxicity in HIV/hepatitis C virus-coinfected patients during interferon plus ribavirin-based therapy. J Acquir Immune Defic Syndr 1999;40(1):47–52.

25. Bani-Sadr F, Goderel I, Penalba C, et al. Risk factors for anaemia in human immunodeficiency virus/hepatitis C virus-coinfected patients treated with interferon plus ribavirin. J Viral Hepat 2007;14(9):639–44.

26. Sulkowski M, Pol S, Mallolas J, et al. Boceprevir versus placebo with pegylated interferon alfa-2b and ribavirin for treatment of hepatitis C virus genotype 1 in patients with HIV: a randomised, double-blind, controlled phase 2 trial. Lancet Infect Dis 2013;13(7):597–605.

27. Sulkowski MS, Sherman KE, Dieterich DT, et al. Combination therapy with telaprevir for chronic hepatitis C virus genotype 1 infection in patients with HIV: a randomized trial. Ann Intern Med 2013;159(2):86–96.

28. Dieterich D, Rockstroh JK, Orkin C, et al. Simeprevir (TMC435) with pegylated interferon/ribavirin in patients coinfected with HCV genotype 1 and HIV-1: a phase 3 study. Clin Infect Dis 2014;59(11):1579–87.

29. Rodriguez-Torres M, Gaggar A, Shen G, et al. Sofosbuvir for chronic hepatitis C virus infection genotype 1-4 in patients co-infected with HIV. J Acquir Immune Defic Syndr 2015;68(5):543–9.

30. Cachay ER, Wyles DL, Torriani FJ, et al. High incidence of serious adverse events in HIV-infected patients treated with a telaprevir-based hepatitis C virus treatment regimen. AIDS Lond Engl 2013;27(18):2893–7.

31. HIV/AIDS treatment guidelines [Internet]. AIDSinfo. Available at: http://aidsinfo.nih.gov/. Accessed July 15, 2015.

32. Günthard HF, Aberg JA, Eron JJ, et al. Antiretroviral treatment of adult HIV infection: 2014 recommendations of the International Antiviral Society–USA Panel. JAMA 2014;312(4):410–25.

33. Bräu N, Salvatore M, Ríos-Bedoya CF, et al. Slower fibrosis progression in HIV/HCV-coinfected patients with successful HIV suppression using antiretroviral therapy. J Hepatol 2006;44(1):47–55.

34. Qurishi N, Kreuzberg C, Lüchters G, et al. Effect of antiretroviral therapy on liver-related mortality in patients with HIV and hepatitis C virus coinfection. Lancet 2003;362(9397):1708–13.

35. Thein H-H, Yi Q, Dore GJ, et al. Natural history of hepatitis C virus infection in HIV-infected individuals and the impact of HIV in the era of highly active antiretroviral therapy: a meta-analysis. AIDS Lond Engl 2008;22(15):1979–91.

36. Sulkowski MS, Mehta SH, Torbenson MS, et al. Rapid fibrosis progression among HIV/hepatitis C virus-co-infected adults. AIDS Lond Engl 2007;21(16):2209–16.

37. Gilead Sciences. SOVALDI® (sofosbuvir) tablets, for oral use. [Internet]. 2014. Available at: https://www.gilead.com/~/media/Files/pdfs/medicines/liver-disease/sovaldi/sovaldi_pi.pdf. Accessed January 30, 2015.

38. Sulkowski MS, Naggie S, Lalezari J, et al. Sofosbuvir and ribavirin for hepatitis C in patients with HIV coinfection. JAMA 2014;312(4):353–61.

39. Molina J-M, Orkin C, Iser D, et al. All-oral therapy with sofosbuvir plus ribavirin for the treatment of HCV genotypes 1, 2, 3 and 4 infection in patients coinfected with HIV (PHOTON-2). Melbourne (Australia). 2014. p. abstract MOAB0105LB. Available at: http://pag.aids2014.org/Abstracts.aspx?SID=1143&AID=11072. Accessed January 30, 2015.

40. Lawitz E, Mangia A, Wyles D, et al. Sofosbuvir for previously untreated chronic hepatitis C infection. N Engl J Med 2013;368(20):1878–87.

41. Jacobson IM, Gordon SC, Kowdley KV, et al. Sofosbuvir for hepatitis C genotype 2 or 3 in patients without treatment options. N Engl J Med 2013;368(20):1867–77.

42. Zeuzem S, Dusheiko GM, Salupere R, et al. Sofosbuvir and ribavirin in HCV genotypes 2 and 3. N Engl J Med 2014;370(21):1993–2001.

43. Kirby B, Mathias A, Rossi S. No clinically significant pharmacokinetic drug interactions between sofosbuvir (GS-7977) and HIV antiretrovirals Atripla,

rilpivirine, darunavir/ritonavir, or raltegravir in healthy volunteers. Hepatology 2012;56(suppl):1067A.

44. Gilead Sciences. HARVONI® (ledipasvir and sofosbuvir) tablets, for oral use [Internet]. 2014. Available at: http://www.gilead.com/~/media/Files/pdfs/medicines/liver-disease/harvoni/harvoni_pi.pdf. Accessed March 23, 2015.

45. Naggie S, Cooper C, Saag M, et al. ION-4 Investigators. Ledipasvir and Sofosbuvir for HCV in Patients Coinfected with HIV-1. N Engl J Med 2015. [Epub ahead of print].

46. Townsend K, Osinusi A, Nelson A, et al. High efficacy of sofosbuvir/ledipasvir for the treatment of HCV genotype 1 in patients coinfected with HIV on or off antiretroviral therapy: results from the NIAID ERADICATE Trial. Hepatology 2014;60:240A–1A.

47. Gao M, Nettles RE, Belema M, et al. Chemical genetics strategy identifies an HCV NS5A inhibitor with a potent clinical effect. Nature [Internet]. 2010. [cited 2010 Apr 26]. http://dx.doi.org/10.1038/nature08960.

48. Bifano M, Hwang C, Oosterhuis B, et al. Assessment of pharmacokinetic interactions of the HCV NS5A replication complex inhibitor daclatasvir with antiretroviral agents: ritonavir-boosted atazanavir, efavirenz and tenofovir. Antivir Ther 2013; 18(7):931–40.

49. Bristol-Myers Squibb. Daklinza 30 mg film-coated tablets [Internet]. 2014. Available at: http://www.ema.europa.eu/docs/en_GB/document_library/EPAR_-_Product_Information/human/003768/WC500172848.pdf.

50. Afdhal N, Zeuzem S, Kwo P, et al. Ledipasvir and sofosbuvir for untreated HCV genotype 1 infection. N Engl J Med 2014;370(20):1889–98.

51. Afdhal N, Reddy KR, Nelson DR, et al. Ledipasvir and sofosbuvir for previously treated HCV genotype 1 infection. N Engl J Med 2014;370(16):1483–93.

52. Sulkowski MS, Gardiner DF, Rodriguez-Torres M, et al. Daclatasvir plus sofosbuvir for previously treated or untreated chronic HCV infection. N Engl J Med 2014; 370(3):211–21.

53. Wyles DL, Ruane PJ, Sulkowski MS, et al. ALLY-2 Investigators. Daclatasvir plus Sofosbuvir for HCV in Patients Coinfected with HIV-1. N Engl J Med 2015. [Epub ahead of print].

54. German P, Pang PS, West S, et al. Drug interactions between direct-acting anti-HCV antivirals sofosbuvir and ledipasvir and HIV antiretrovirals. Washington, DC: 2014.

55. Gilead Sciences. VIREAD® (tenofovir disoproxil fumarate) tablets, for oral use [Internet]. 2013. Available at: http://www.gilead.com/~/media/Files/pdfs/medicines/liver-disease/viread/viread_pi.pdf. Accessed January 30, 2015.

56. Weiss J, Herzog M, König S, et al. Induction of multiple drug transporters by efavirenz. J Pharmacol Sci 2009 Feb;109(2):242–50.

57. Eley T, You X, Wang R, et al. Daclatasvir: overview of drug-drug interactions with antiretroviral agents and other common concomitant drugs. Miami (FL): 2014.

58. Janssen Therapeutics. OLYSIO (simeprevir) capsules, for oral use. [Internet]. 2014. Available at: https://www.olysio.com/shared/product/olysio/prescribing-information.pdf. Accessed January 30, 2015.

59. Lawitz E, Sulkowski MS, Ghalib R, et al. Simeprevir plus sofosbuvir, with or without ribavirin, to treat chronic infection with hepatitis C virus genotype 1 in non-responders to pegylated interferon and ribavirin and treatment-naive patients: the COSMOS randomised study. Lancet 2014;384(9956):1756–65.

60. Ouwerkerk-Mahadevan S, Sekar V, Simion A, et al. The pharmacokinetic interactions of the HCV protease inhibitor simeprevir (TMC435) with HIV antiretroviral agents in healthy volunteers. San Diego (CA): 2012.

61. AbbVie Inc. VIEKIRA PAK (ombitasvir, paritaprevir, and ritonavir tablets; dasabuvir tablets), co-packaged for oral use. [Internet]. 2014. Available at: http://www.rxabbvie.com/pdf/viekirapak_pi.pdf. Accessed March 23, 2015.

62. Sulkowski MS, Eron JJ, Wyles D, et al. Ombitasvir, paritaprevir co-dosed with ritonavir, dasabuvir, and ribavirin for hepatitis C in patients co-infected with HIV-1: a randomized trial. JAMA 2015;313(12):1223–31.

63. Khatri A, Wang T, Wang H. Drug-drug interactions of the direct acting antiviral regimen of ABT-450/r, ombitasvir and dasabuvir with HIV protease inhibitors [abstract V-484]. Washington, DC; 2014.

64. Khatri A, Wang T, Wang H. Drug-drug interactions of the direct acting antiviral regimen ofABT-450/r, ombitasvir and dasabuvir with emtricitabine + tenofovir, raltegravir, rilpivirine and efavirenz [abstract V-483]. Washington, DC; 2014.

65. Janssen Therapeutics. EDURANT (rilpivirine) tablets for oral use [Internet]. 2014. Available at: http://www.edurant.com/sites/default/files/EDURANT-PI.pdf. Accessed January 30, 2015.

66. McKeage K, Perry CM, Keam SJ. Darunavir: a review of its use in the management of HIV infection in adults. Drugs 2009;69(4):477–503.

67. Eron JJ, Young B, Cooper DA, et al. Switch to a raltegravir-based regimen versus continuation of a lopinavir-ritonavir-based regimen in stable HIV-infected patients with suppressed viraemia (SWITCHMRK 1 and 2): two multicentre, double-blind, randomised controlled trials. Lancet 2010;375(9712):396–407.

68. Llibre JM, Pulido F, García F, et al. Genetic barrier to resistance for dolutegravir. AIDS Rev 2014;17(1):56–64.

69. Rathbun RC, Lockhart SM, Miller MM, et al. Dolutegravir, a second-generation integrase inhibitor for the treatment of HIV-1 infection. Ann Pharmacother 2014; 48(3):395–403.

70. Castagna A, Maggiolo F, Penco G, et al. Dolutegravir in antiretroviral-experienced patients with raltegravir- and/or elvitegravir-resistant HIV-1: 24-week results of the phase III VIKING-3 study. J Infect Dis 2014;210(3):354–62.

71. Turriziani O, Andreoni M, Antonelli G. Resistant viral variants in cellular reservoirs of human immunodeficiency virus infection. Clin Microbiol Infect 2010 Oct;16(10): 1518–24.

72. HCV policy & advocacy [Internet]. HIVandHepatitis.com. Available at: http://www.hivandhepatitis.com/hcv-policy-advocacy/4837-community-leaders-hiv-doctors-oppose-hepatitis-c-treatment-barriers. Accessed February 4, 2015.

73. American Academy of HIV Medicine and HIV Medicine Association. HIV medical organizations challenge insurer restrictions to HCV treatment. [Internet]. 2014. Available at: http://www.hivma.org/AAHIVM_HIVMA/. Accessed January 30, 2015.

74. Infectious Diseases Society of America and HIV Medicine Association. IDSA, HIVMA call for state Medicaid programs to lift hepatitis C prescribing restrictions from ID and HIV doctors. [Internet]. 2014. Available at: http://www.idsociety.org/HCV_Provider_Restrictions/. Accessed January 30, 2015.

Next-Generation Regimens
The Future of Hepatitis C Virus Therapy

John Vizuete, MD, MPH*, Hope Hubbard, MD, Eric Lawitz, MD

KEYWORDS

- Hepatitis C • Genotype 1 • Direct-acting antivirals • Second generation
- Resistance-associated variants

KEY POINTS

- The rapid developments in therapy for hepatitis C have been historic, and have ushered in a new paradigm for the treatment of hepatitis C.
- Although prior therapeutic regimens were limited by efficacy, tolerability, genotype specificity, and duration of therapy, numerous improved agents are in development.
- Optimal combinations should facilitate a fixed duration of therapy for all patient subtypes.

INTRODUCTION

The treatment of chronic hepatitis C virus (HCV) has undergone a recent phase of rapid evolution. At the present time, 3 interferon (IFN)-free direct-acting antiviral (DAA) regimens are approved for the treatment of HCV genotype 1. Within the next few years, continued development of novel agents and combinations is expected, with the aim of coming closer to the ideal regimen. This article focuses on future therapeutic options for HCV with an emphasis on drug development and key ongoing trials.

LIMITATIONS OF PAST REGIMENS

Prior to the DAA era, HCV treatment was limited by the adverse effect profile and poor efficacy of IFN/ribavirin (RBV)-based regimens. Although the advent of DAAs has

Disclosures: Dr E. Lawitz has received research and grant support from AbbVie, Achillion Pharmaceuticals, Boehringer Ingelheim, Bristol-Myers Squibb, Gilead Sciences, GlaxoSmithKline, Idenix Pharmaceuticals, Janssen, Merck & Co., Novartis, Presidio, Roche, Salix, Santaris Pharmaceuticals, Theravance, and Vertex Pharmaceuticals. He has also served as a speaker for AbbVie, Gilead, Janssen, and has provided advisory and consultation services to AbbVie, Achillion Pharmaceuticals, BioCryst, Biotica, Bristol-Myers Squibb, Enanta, Gilead Sciences, Idenix Pharmaceuticals, Janssen, Merck & Co., Novartis, Santaris Pharmaceuticals, Regulus, Theravance, and Vertex Pharmaceuticals. Dr J. Vizuete and Dr H. Hubbard have nothing to disclose.
Division of Gastroenterology and Nutrition, Department of Medicine, University of Texas Health Science Center at San Antonio, 7703 Floyd Curl Drive, San Antonio, TX 78229, USA
* Corresponding author.
E-mail address: johnvizuete@gmail.com

Clin Liver Dis 19 (2015) 707–716
http://dx.doi.org/10.1016/j.cld.2015.06.009
1089-3261/15/$ – see front matter © 2015 Elsevier Inc. All rights reserved.

liver.theclinics.com

brought marked improvements in tolerability and efficacy, current therapies remain limited by variable durations of therapy ranging from 8 to 24 weeks and genotype specificity. Future regimens should target these limitations.

PHASE III TRIALS
Daclatasvir/Asunaprevir/Beclabuvir

Phase III data for another oral DAA regimen expected to reach the US market have been reported. Combination daclatasvir (30 mg daily), asunaprevir (200 mg daily), and beclabuvir (75 mg daily) in a twice-daily fixed dose (DCV-TRIO) was administered to 415 treatment naïve and experienced (pegylated interferon [PEG-IFN]/RBV), noncirrhotic genotype patients for 12 weeks, dubbed UNITY-I.[1] SVR12 was comparable for treatment-naïve and experienced patients (91% vs 89% respectively) regardless of baseline HCV RNA level or interleukin (IL)28 b genotype. When stratified by subgenotype, G1b patients were more likely to achieve SVR than G1a patients regardless of prior treatment exposure (98% vs 90% for naïve patients and 100% vs 85% for experienced patients). This study did not include RBV; however, one of the currently approved regimens that includes a protease inhibitor, NS5A inhibitor, and non-nucleotide polymerase inhibitor demonstrated superior rates of SVR (90% vs 96%) in G1a patients when RBV was included.[2] DCV-TRIO was well tolerated, with the most common adverse events being headache (26%), fatigue (17%), diarrhea (14%), and nausea (13%). Alanine aminotransferase (ALT) elevation was reported in 5% of patients and led to discontinuation in 2 cases.

UNITY-II examined the same drug combination plus or minus RBV for 12 weeks in genotype 1 patients with compensated Child-Pugh class A cirrhosis.[3] SVR12 rates of 93% and 87% were seen in naïve and experienced patients, respectively, with DCV-TRIO alone. When RBV was included for G1a patients, SVR12 increased to 98% and 93%. The most commonly reported adverse events included headache (17%), nausea (14%), diarrhea (13%), and fatigue (12%). Fatigue and headache increased to 28% and 23%, respectively, when RBV was included. Three out of 202 patients discontinued therapy because of adverse events, 2 because of anemia and 1 because of anemia and increased aspartate aminotransferase (AST), all in the RBV group. DCV-TRIO has the opportunity to enter the competitive genotype 1 market in which more therapeutic options for physicians should only enhance patient care.

Daclatasvir/Sofosbuvir

The ALLY-3 trial combines daclatasvir (60 mg daily) with sofosbuvir (400 mg daily) for G3 patients in an open-label 12-week trial.[4] This regimen has previously demonstrated excellent efficacy in G1-3 with a 24-week duration.[5] Currently the only IFN-free therapy for G3 is sofosbuvir and RBV for a 24-week duration; this therapy has demonstrated higher rates of SVR (60%–94%) compared with 12- or 16-week durations.[6,7] Durations of 12 to 16 weeks in treatment-naïve patients had SVR rates of 55%, while treatment-experienced patients had SVR rates of 36% to 62%. IFN-ineligible patients treated for 12 weeks had overall SVR rates of 61%, 21% for cirrhotic patients and 68% for noncirrhotic patients. Treatment-experienced cirrhotic patients are not optimally served by this regimen, with SVR12 rates 19% to 60% with 12- to 16-week durations, respectively.[8] ALLY-3 examined SVR in treatment-naïve and -experienced cirrhotic and noncirrhotic patients. SVR rates of 97% and 94% were seen in noncirrhotic naïve and experienced patients, respectively. The presence of cirrhosis reduced SVR to 58% and 69%. The combination was well tolerated, with infrequent reported adverse effects of headache (20%), fatigue (18%), nausea (12%), and diarrhea (9%). No treatment-related serious adverse events were seen. This study supports a shorter, RBV-free regimen for G3 patients. However, future regimens are anticipated that can produce high rates of SVR in G3 patients irrespective of the presence or absence of cirrhosis.

PHASE II TRIALS
Grazoprevir (MK-5172)/Elbasvir (MK-8742)

Results from the C-WORTHY trial have been published and have examined the use of grazoprevir, an NS3/4A protease inhibitor and elbasvir, an NS5A inhibitor with and without RBV for G1 patients. C-WORTHY evaluated both treatment-naïve patients with or without human immunodeficiency virus (HIV) coinfection[9] in addition to traditionally more difficult-to-treat patients including those with cirrhosis and previous null response, with or without cirrhosis.[10]

Sulkowski and colleagues randomized monoinfected treatment-naïve patients to either 8 weeks (genotype 1a only) of grazoprevir (100 mg daily), elbasvir (50 mg daily) and RBV or 12 weeks of grazoprevir (100 mg daily) and elbasvir (50 mg daily) with or without RBV (genotype 1a or 1b). The 8-week group had an SVR12 of 80%, while the 12-week groups had SVR12 rates of 93% and 98%, with or without RBV. Coinfected treatment-naïve patients had similar rates of SVR12 with a 12-week duration of therapy, with rates of 97% and 87% with or without RBV.

Lawitz and colleagues evaluated treatment-naïve patients with cirrhosis and null responders with or without cirrhosis with grazoprevir and elbasvir with or without RBV for 12 or 18 weeks.

High SVR rates were seen in all groups (90%–100%), and extending therapy to 18 weeks did not confer additional benefit for any group. Overall SVR rates of 94% and 95% were seen in naïve and prior null responders, respectively. RBV therapy did not influence SVR (95% + RBV vs 94% -RBV). Cirrhotic patients and noncirrhotic patients had the same overall SVR of 95%.

Reported adverse effects included fatigue (26%), headache (23%), and weakness (14%). Serious adverse events were rare. Patients taking RBV-containing regimens demonstrated anemia (12%) and elevation in total bilirubin greater than 2.5 times baseline (12%), which did not occur in the RBV-free arms. The overall high efficacy rates in prior null responders and cirrhotic patients provides the potential for a fixed duration for patients irrespective of the presence or absence of cirrhosis; however, phase III results are awaited to confirm the phase II findings.

HCV monoinfected patients treated for 8 weeks with RBV had SVR12 rates of 80% (24/30). Monoinfected patients treated for 12 weeks with and without RBV showed SVR12 of 93% (79/85) and 98% (43/44), respectively. HIV/HCV coinfected patients treated for 12 weeks with and without RBV had response rates of 97% (28/29) and 87% (26/30), respectively. In these groups, there were no discontinuations due to adverse events or laboratory abnormality. The most common adverse events were fatigue (23%), headache (20%), nausea (15%), and diarrhea (10%).

One approach to decrease duration of therapy while maintaining high SVR is to combine multiple potent DAAs with a high barrier to resistance and unique mechanisms of action. In a proof-of-concept study, C-SWIFT, the combination of sofusbuvir, grazoprevir and elbasvir, was evaluated with a short duration of therapy.[11] Noncirrhotic G1 patients were treated for either 4 or 6 weeks, while cirrhotic patients were treated for 6 or 8 weeks.

SVR 4/8 was 39% in the 4-week, noncirrhotic group, but this improved to 87% with 6 weeks of treatment. SVR4/8 in cirrhotic patients was 80% in the 6-week group and

95% (18/19) in the 8-week group. The regimen was well tolerated with low rates of adverse events in all groups. C-SWIFT demonstrates that treatment durations as short as 4 weeks are biologically plausible, but further improvements in potency of DAA therapy are needed to make this short-duration therapy more universally successful.

GS-5816/Sofosbuvir

Data are now available for the GS-5816, a pan-genotypic NS5A inhibitor in a fixed dose combination with sofosbuvir. Everson and colleagues[12] have reported highly successful cure rates after 12 weeks of therapy in G1-G6 patients. Patients were randomized to 25 mg or 100 mg GS-5816 plus 400 mg sofosbuvir. Of 154 patients in this intent-to-treat analysis, there were only 4 treatment failures across all genotypes (SVR = 97%). SVR rates by genotype in the 25 mg group are as follows: G1 96% (26/27), G2 91% (10/11), G3 93% (25/27), G4 100% (7/7), G5 100% (1/1), and G6 100% (4/4). In the 100 mg group, rates by genotype were: G1 100% (28/28), G2 100% (10/10), G3 93% (25/27), G4 86% (6/7), and G6 100% (5/5). The most frequent adverse events were fatigue (21%), headache (19%), and nausea (12%), with no serious treatment-related adverse events and no significant laboratory abnormalities.

In a second phase, the same regimen was tested with and without RBV in an 8-week regimen in genotypes 1–3.[13] SVR rates by genotype were numerically lower with this duration of therapy, ranging from 77% to 90% with 8 weeks of treatment compared to 91%–100% with 12 weeks of treatment. Adverse effect profiles were similar. To optimize rates of SVR, a 12-week duration should be further investigated, and if these results are validated in phase III, it would offer the first pan-genotypic fixed-dose combination tablet with comparable rates of SVR across genotypes.

ACH-3102

In phase I studies, ACH-3102, an NS5A inhibitor, has demonstrated high in vitro potency against multiple resistance-associated variants (RAVs).[14] A small phase II trial combined ACH-3102 with sofosbuvir.[15] Twelve treatment-naïve, noncirrhotic G1 patients received 50 mg ACH-3102 and 400 mg sofosbuvir for 8 weeks. All 12 patients exhibited SVR at follow-up week 12. Interim top line results from a similar 6-week trial have since been released, indicating 100% SVR in a separate 12-patient cohort. SVR was attained regardless of viral load or IL28b status.[16] This regimen was well tolerated, without any early treatment discontinuations. Given these results, larger trials across more diverse patient populations should be undertaken. A comparison of phase II and III trials may be found in **Table 1**.

PHASE I
ABT-493/ABT-530

ABT-493 is a second-generation protease inhibitor, and ABT-530 is a second-generation NS5A inhibitor. Both are potent, pan-genotypic agents with high barriers to resistance. Both of these agents demonstrated a greater than 4 log decline in viral load regardless of the presence or absence of cirrhosis in a 3-day dose-ranging study of 89 G1 patients.[17] Common adverse effects included headache (22%), abdominal discomfort (6%), and diarrhea (6%) for ABT-493 and headache (10%) and constipation (5%) for ABT-530. Results of these agents in combination direct antiviral regimens are anticipated.

MK-3682 (Formally IDX21437)

MK-3682 is a nucleotide NS5B polymerase inhibitor with potent pharmacokinetics and pan-genotypic activity. Phase I testing showed mean maximal viral load reductions of

Table 1
Summary of phase II and III trials

Study	Regimen	Patients	Genotype	N	SVR 12
ACH-3102	ACH 3102 Sofosbuvir	Treatment-naïve noncirrhotic	1	24 patients	100%
C-SWIFT	Grazoprevir Elbasvir Sofosbuvir	Treatment-naïve with and without cirrhosis	1	102 patients	SVR 4/8 Noncirrhotic 4 wk: 38.7% 6 wk: 86.7% Cirrhosis 6 wk: 80% 8 wk: 94.7%
C-WORTHY – 12 wk	Grazoprevir Elbasvir +/– RBV	Treatment-naïve with cirrhosis Treatment-experienced with and without cirrhosis	1	125 patients	Treatment-naïve cirrhosis + RBV: 90% Treatment-naïve cirrhosis without RBV: 97% Treatment-experienced + RBV: 94% Treatment-experienced without RBV: 91%
C-WORTHY – 18 wk	Grazoprevir Elbasvir +/– RBV	Treatment-naïve with cirrhosis Treatment-experienced with and without cirrhosis	1	128 patients	Treatment-naïve cirrhosis + RBV: 97% Treatment-naïve cirrhosis without RBV: 94% Treatment-experienced + RBV: 100% Treatment-experienced without RBV: 97%
C-WORTHY – HIV co-infected	Grazoprevir Elbasvir	Treatment-naïve, non-cirrhotic monoinfected and HIV coinfected	1	218 patients	HIV coinfected + RBV: 97% HIV coinfected without RBV: 87% Monoinfected + RBV: 93% Monoinfected without RBV: 98%
ALLY-3	Daclatasvir Sofosbuvir	Treatment-naïve and treatment-experienced with and without cirrhosis	3	152 patients	Treatment-naïve noncirrhotic: 97% Treatment-naïve cirrhotic: 58% Treatment-experienced noncirrhotic: 94% Treatment-experienced cirrhotic patients: 69%

(continued on next page)

Table 1
(continued)

Study	Regimen	Patients	Genotype	N	SVR 12
UNITY-1	Daclatasvir Asunaprevir Beclabuvir	Treatment-naïve and treatment-experienced noncirrhotic patients	1	415 patients	Treatment-naïve: 92% Treatment-experienced: 89%
UNITY-2	Daclatasvir Asunaprevir Beclabuvir +/− RBV	Treatment-naïve and treatment-experienced with cirrhosis	1	202 patients	Treatment-naïve + RBV: 98% Treatment-naïve without RBV: 93% Treatment-experienced + RBV: 93% Treatment-experienced without RBV: 87%
GS-5816	GS-5816 (100 mg) Sofosbuvir	Treatment-naïve noncirrhotic	1–6	154 patients	Genotypes 1–2: 100% Genotype 3: 93% Genotype 4: 86% Genotype 5: N/A Genotype 6: 100%

4.8 and 3.9 log for G1a/1b and 4.6 and 4.1 log reductions in G2/3 with 7-days of 300 mg/d dosing.[18] It was well tolerated without any significant laboratory findings. Phase II studies are planned to evaluate 2 regimens with variable durations: MK-3682 in combination with grazoprevir/elbasvir or grazoprevir/MK8408 (preclinical NS5A inhibitor). Results of these phase 2 trials are awaited.

PRECLINICAL AGENTS
MK-8408

MK-8408 is a potent pan-genotypic NS5A inhibitor that exhibits activity against key resistance-associated variants, Q30R and Y93H, which are common treatment emergent variants that appear after failure of a current NS5A inhibitor-based therapy.[19] It has a high genetic barrier to resistance, and its kinetics support daily dosing. Additionally, in vitro studies with MK-8408 and grazoprevir demonstrate an additive and possibly synergistic interaction with an improved clinical profile over elbasvir, particularly in G3 patients.[20] The authors look forward to clinical data with MK 8408 in combination with other antivirals.

HOST TARGETED AGENTS

In addition to targeting viral encoded proteins, there is potential for drug development aimed at the host, known as host targeting agents (HTAs). A novel class of HTAs is based on the fact that HCV is protected within the hepatocyte by an abundant liver-specific microRNA (miRNA) called miR-122.[21] miR-122 binds to 2 highly conserved sites (s1 and s2) of the HCV genome, preventing recognition and degradation by host enzymes.[22] miR-122 seed sequences are highly conserved across all HCV genotypes and are thus inherently pan-genotypic, with no reported RAVs. Agents targeting miR-122 are dosed percutaneously.[23] The most significant historical limitation to HTA development has been the systemic effects of therapy. There may be opportunities in the future to combine a well-tolerated HTA and DAA(s) to shorten courses of therapy yet continue to achieve high rates of SVR. This approach will only be practical if one can shorten duration yet still achieve the same rates of SVR with no additional adverse events. No studies have reported outcomes of combining MiR-122 inhibitors with DAA therapy.

MIRAVIRSEN

Miravirsen is an injectable complimentary 15-nucleotide chain that binds to and inhibits miR-122 and has been studied in 36 noncirrhotic genotype 1 patients in a dose-ranging study.[24] They observed a dose-dependent reduction in HCV RNA levels with weekly dosing for 5 weeks. After 14 weeks, 1 patient in the 5 mg group and 4 patients in the 7 mg group exhibited persistent HCV undetectability. Persistent undetectability was seen in 60% of those receiving 3 mg/kg miravirsen, 25% of those receiving 5 mg/kg miraversen, and 100% of those receiving 7 mg/kg miraversen. Adverse events were reported 4 times as often in the miravirsen group compared with the placebo group and included headache (22%–44%), fatigue (11%–33%), and injection site reactions (2 of 9 patients in the 7 mg group). Follow-up data at 35 months revealed no significant longer-term treatment-related adverse events, hospitalizations, or deaths.[25]

RG-101

RG-101 is a miR-122 inhibitor with potent in vitro activity that is currently being studied in a single-dose, dose-ranging trial. Interim results from a phase IIa study comparing a single administration of either 2 mg or 4 mg have shown 9 of 14 (64%) patients in the 4 mg group with HCV RNA less than 15 IU/mL at 8 weeks compared to 6 of 14 patients (43%) in the 2 mg group.[26] Full safety and efficacy results are expected in 2015. The prolonged biologic effects after a single dose warrant future trials to coadminister RG-101 with DAA therapy with the goal of shortening treatment duration.

FUTURE FRONTIERS

The race to develop the optimal regimen is far from over. Vigorous development plans continue to emerge. There continues to be hope of finding a pan-genotypic regimen that delivers high rates of SVR across all genotypes and populations. Today, factors including the presence/absence of cirrhosis, genotype/subtype, baseline viral load, and previous treatment experience affect the duration of therapy, which currently ranges from 8 to 24 weeks. Optimal combinations should facilitate a fixed duration of therapy for all patient subtypes. C-SWIFT demonstrates that a fixed 8-week duration is an achievable target; in addition, the trial demonstrated the biologic plausibility of durations as short as 4 weeks. Comparable low rates of relapse will need to be demonstrated before short durations of therapy become the standard of care. To achieve this goal, a new generation of antivirals may be required. New data are awaited that will bring closer the ideal regimen that would deliver high rates of SVR (>95%) across all genotypes and be agnostic to previous treatment experience and the presence or absence of cirrhosis.

The rapid developments in therapy for hepatitis C have been historic and have ushered in a new paradigm for the treatment of hepatitis C. The authors look forward to future developments that will bring the optimal regimen closer with the ultimate goal of eradicating hepatitis C from the world.

REFERENCES

1. Poordad F, Sievert W, Mollison L, et al. All-oral, fixed-dose combination therapy with daclatasvir/asunaprevir/beclabuvir for non-cirrhotic patients with chronic HCV genotype 1 infection: UNITY-1 phase 3 SVR-12 results [LB-7]. Presented at the 65th Annual Meeting of the American Association for the Study of Liver Diseases. Boston, November 10, 2014.
2. Ferenci P, Bernstein D, Lalezari J, et al. ABT-450/r-ombitasvir and dasabuvir with or without ribavirin for HCV. N Engl J Med 2014;370:1983–92.
3. Muir AJ, Poordad F, Lalezari J, et al. All-oral, fixed-dose combination therapy with daclatasvir/asunaprevir/beclabuvir ± ribavirin, for patients with chronic HCV genotype 1 infection and compensated cirrhosis: UNITY-2 phase 3 SVR12 results [LB-2]. Presented at the 65th Annual Meeting of the American Association for the Study of Liver Diseases. Boston, November 10, 2014.
4. Nelson DR, Cooper JN, Lalezari JP, et al. All-oral 12-week combination treatment with daclatasvir (DCV) and sofosbuvir (SOF) in patients infected with HCV genotype (GT) 3: ALLY-3 phase 3 study [LB-2]. Presented at the 65th Annual Meeting of the American Association for the Study of Liver Diseases. Boston, November 9, 2014.
5. Sulkowski MS, Gardiner DF, Rodriguez-Torres M, et al. Daclatasvir plus sofosbuvir for previously treated or untreated chronic HCV infection. N Engl J Med 2014; 370:211–21.
6. Zeuzem S, Dusheiko GM, Salupere R, et al. Sofosbuvir and ribavirin in HCV genotypes 2 and 3. N Engl J Med 2014;370:1993–2001.

7. Lawitz E, Mangia A, Wyles D, et al. Sofosbuvir for previously untreated chronic hepatitis C infection. N Engl J Med 2013;368:1878–87.
8. Jacobson IM, Gordon SC, Kowdley KV, et al. Sofosbuvir for hepatitis C genotype 2 or 3 in patients without treatment options. N Engl J Med 2013;368:1867–77.
9. Sulkowski M, Hezode C, Gerstoft J, et al. Efficacy and safety of 8 weeks versus 12 weeks of treatment with grazoprevir (MK-5172) and elbasvir (MK-8742) with or without ribavirin in patients with hepatitis C virus genotype 1 mono-infection and HIV/hepatitis C virus co-infection (C-WORTHY): a randomised, open-label phase 2 trial. Lancet 2014;385:1087–97.
10. Lawitz E, Gane E, Pearlman B, et al. Efficacy and safety of 12 weeks versus 18 weeks of treatment with grazoprevir (MK-5172) and elbasvir (MK-8742) with or without ribavirin for hepatitis C virus genotype 1 infection in previously untreated patients with cirrhosis and patients with previous null response with or without cirrhosis (C-WORTHY): a randomised, open-label phase 2 trial. Lancet 2014; 385:1075–86.
11. Lawitz E, Poordad F, Gutierrez JA, et al. C-SWIFT: grazoprevir (MK-5172)+ elbasvir (MK-8742)+ sofosbuvir in treatment-naive patients with hepatitis C virus genotype 1 infection, with and without cirrhosis, for durations of 4, 6, or 8 weeks (interim Results) [LB-33]. Presented at the 65th Annual Meeting of the American Association for the Study of Liver Diseases. Boston, November 9, 2014.
12. Everson GT, Tran TT, Towner WJ, et al. Safety and efficacy of treatment with the interferon-free, ribavirin-free combination of sofosbuvir+ Gs-5816 for 12 weeks in treatment naive patients with genotype 1–6 HCV infection [abstract 111]. Presented at the 49th annual meeting of the European Association for the Study of the Liver. London, April 11, 2014.
13. Tran TT, Morgan TR, Thuluvath PJ, et al. Safety and Efficacy of treatment with sofosbuvir+ GS-5816+/− ribavirin for 8 or 12 weeks in treatment naive patients with genotype 1-6 HCV infection [abstract: 80]. Presented at the 65th Annual Meeting of the American Association for the Study of Liver Diseases. Boston, November 9, 2014.
14. Muir A, Hill J, Lawitz E, et al. ACH-3102, a second generation NS5A inhibitor, demonstrates potent antiviral activity in patients with genotype 1a HCV infection despite the presence of baseline NS5A-resistant variants [abstract 398]. Presented at the 48th annual meeting of the European Association for the Study of the Liver. Amsterdam, April 27, 2013.
15. Gane EJ, Kocinsky H, Schwabe C, et al. Interim sustained virologic response (SVR), safety and tolerability results of 8-week treatment with ACH-3102 and sofosbuvir in chronic hepatitis C (HCV), genotype-1 (GT-1), treatment-naive patients: a phase 2 "proxy" study [LB-32]. Presented at the 65th Annual Meeting of the American Association for the Study of Liver Diseases. Boston, November 9, 2014.
16. Achillion achieves 100% SVR12 in phase 2 trial evaluating 6-week combination treatment with ACH-3102. 2015. Available at: http://ir.achillion.com/releasedetail.cfm?releaseid=895306. Accessed February 11, 2015.
17. Lawitz E, O'Riordan WD, Freilich BL, et al. Potent antiviral activity of ABT-493 and ABT-530 with 3-day monotherapy in patients with and without compensated cirrhosis with hepatitis C virus (HCV) genotype 1 infection [abstract 1956]. Presented at the 65th Annual Meeting of the American Association for the Study of Liver Diseases. Boston, November 9, 2014.
18. Gane EJ, Sicard E, Popa S, et al. A phase I/IIa study assessing 7-day dosing of MK-3682 (formerly IDX21437) in subjects infected with hepatitis C virus (HCV)

[abstract: 1974]. Presented at the 65th Annual Meeting of the American Association for the Study of Liver Diseases. Boston, November 9, 2014.

19. Asante-Appiah E, Liu R, Curry S, et al. MK-8408, A potent and selective NS5A inhibitor with a high genetic barrier to resistance and activity against HCV genotypes 1–6 [abstract: 1979]. Presented at the 65th Annual Meeting of the American Association for the Study of Liver Diseases. Boston, November 9, 2014.

20. Lahser F, Bystol K, Curry S, et al. The combination of MK-5172, an NS3 inhibitor, and MK-8408, an NS5A inhibitor, presents a high genetic barrier to resistance in HCV genotypes [abstract: 1988]. Presented at the 65th Annual Meeting of the American Association for the Study of Liver Diseases. Boston, November 9, 2014.

21. Jopling CL, Yi M, Lancaster AM, et al. Modulation of hepatitis C virus RNA abundance by a liver-specific microRNA. Science 2005;309:1577–81.

22. Li Z, Rana TM. Therapeutic targeting of microRNAs: current status and future challenges. Nat Rev Drug Discov 2014;13:622–38.

23. Israelow B, Mullokandov G, Agudo J, et al. Hepatitis C virus genetics affects miR-122 requirements and response to miR-122 inhibitors. Nat Commun 2014;18: 5408.

24. Janssen HL, Reesink HW, Lawitz EJ, et al. Treatment of HCV infection by targeting microRNA. N Engl J Med 2013;368:1685–94.

25. Van der Ree MH, Van der Meer AJ, de Bruijne J, et al. Long-term safety and efficacy of microRNA-targeted therapy in chronic hepatitis C patients. Antiviral Res 2014;111:53–9.

26. All HCV patients treated with a single SC administration of 4 mg/kg of RG-101 responded with mean viral load reduction of 4.8 log10 at Day 29 and 9/14 patients are below the limit of quantification at Day 57. 2015. Available at: http://ir.regulusrx.com/releasedetail.cfm?ReleaseID-=895314. Accessed February 11, 2015.

United States Postal Service

Statement of Ownership, Management, and Circulation
(All Periodicals Publications Except Requester Publications)

1. Publication Title	2. Publication Number	3. Filing Date
Clinics in Liver Disease	0 1 6 - 7 5 4	9/18/15

4. Issue Frequency	5. Number of Issues Published Annually	6. Annual Subscription Price
Feb, May, Aug, Nov	4	$295.00

7. Complete Mailing Address of Known Office of Publication (Not printer) (Street, city, county, state, and ZIP+4®)

Elsevier Inc.
360 Park Avenue South
New York, NY 10010-1710

Contact Person
Stephen R. Bushing

Telephone (Include area code)
215-239-3688

8. Complete Mailing Address of Headquarters or General Business Office of Publisher (Not printer)

Elsevier Inc., 360 Park Avenue South, New York, NY 10010-1710

9. Full Names and Complete Mailing Addresses of Publisher, Editor, and Managing Editor (Do not leave blank)

Publisher (Name and complete mailing address)

Linda Belfus, Elsevier Inc., 1600 John F. Kennedy Blvd., Suite 1800, Philadelphia, PA 19103

Editor (Name and complete mailing address)

Kerry Holland, Elsevier Inc., 1600 John F. Kennedy Blvd., Suite 1800, Philadelphia, PA 19103-2899

Managing Editor (Name and complete mailing address)

Adrianne Brigido, Elsevier Inc., 1600 John F. Kennedy Blvd., Suite 1800, Philadelphia, PA 19103-2899

10. Owner (Do not leave blank. If the publication is owned by a corporation, give the name and address of the corporation immediately followed by the names and addresses of all stockholders owning or holding 1 percent or more of the total amount of stock. If not owned by a corporation, give the names and addresses of the individual owners. If owned by a partnership or other unincorporated firm, give its name and address as well as those of each individual owner. If the publication is published by a nonprofit organization, give its name and address.)

Full Name	Complete Mailing Address
Wholly owned subsidiary of	1600 John F. Kennedy Blvd, Ste. 1800
Reed/Elsevier, US holdings	Philadelphia, PA 19103-2899

11. Known Bondholders, Mortgagees, and Other Security Holders Owning or Holding 1 Percent or More of Total Amount of Bonds, Mortgages, or Other Securities. If none, check box   ☐ None

Full Name	Complete Mailing Address
N/A	

12. Tax Status (For completion by nonprofit organizations authorized to mail at nonprofit rates) (Check one)
The purpose, function, and nonprofit status of this organization and the exempt status for federal income tax purposes:
☐ Has Not Changed During Preceding 12 Months
☐ Has Changed During Preceding 12 Months (Publisher must submit explanation of change with this statement)

13. Publication Title	14. Issue Date for Circulation Data Below
Clinics in Liver Disease	August 2015

15. Extent and Nature of Circulation			Average No. Copies Each Issue During Preceding 12 Months	No. Copies of Single Issue Published Nearest to Filing Date
a. Total Number of Copies (Net press run)			410	412
b. Legitimate Paid and/Or Requested Distribution (By Mail and Outside the Mail)	(1)	Mailed Outside County Paid/Requested Mail Subscriptions stated on PS Form 3541. (Include paid distribution above nominal rate, advertiser's proof copies and exchange copies)	111	90
	(2)	Mailed In-County Paid/Requested Mail Subscriptions stated on PS Form 3541. (Include paid distribution above nominal rate, advertiser's proof copies and exchange copies)		
	(3)	Paid Distribution Outside the Mails Including Sales Through Dealers And Carriers, Street Vendors, Counter Sales, and Other Paid Distribution Outside USPS®	74	91
	(4)	Paid Distribution by Other Classes of Mail Through the USPS (e.g. First-Class Mail®)		
c. Total Paid and or Requested Circulation (Sum of 15b (1), (2), (3), and (4))			185	181
d. Free or Nominal Rate Distribution (By Mail and Outside the Mail)	(1)	Free or Nominal Rate Outside-County Copies included on PS Form 3541	78	91
	(2)	Free or Nominal Rate In-County Copies included on PS Form 3541		
	(3)	Free or Nominal Rate Copies mailed at Other classes Through the USPS (e.g. First-Class Mail)		
	(4)	Free or Nominal Rate Distribution Outside the Mail (Carriers or Other means)		
e. Total Nonrequested Distribution (Sum of 15d (1), (2), (3) and (4))			78	91
f. Total Distribution (Sum of 15c and 15e)			263	272
g. Copies not Distributed (See instructions to publishers #4 (page #3))			147	140
h. Total (Sum of 15f and g)			410	412
i. Percent Paid and/or Requested Circulation (15c divided by 15f times 100)			70.34%	66.54%

* If you are claiming electronic copies go to line 16 on page 3. If you are not claiming Electronic copies, skip to line 17 on page 3.

16. Electronic Copy Circulation	Average No. Copies Each Issue During Preceding 12 Months	No. Copies of Single Issue Published Nearest to Filing Date
a. Paid Electronic Copies		
b. Total paid Print Copies (Line 15c) + Paid Electronic copies (Line 16a)		
c. Total Print Distribution (Line 15f) + Paid Electronic Copies (Line 16a)		
d. Percent Paid (Both Print & Electronic copies) (16b divided by 16c X 100)		

☐ I certify that 50% of all my distributed copies (electronic and print) are paid above a nominal price

17. Publication of Statement of Ownership
If the publication is a general publication, publication of this statement is required. Will be printed in the November 2015 issue of this publication.

18. Signature and Title of Editor, Publisher, Business Manager, or Owner

Stephen R. Bushing

Stephen R. Bushing – Inventory Distribution Coordinator

Date
September 18, 2015

I certify that all information furnished on this form is true and complete. I understand that anyone who furnishes false or misleading information on this form or who omits material or information requested on the form may be subject to criminal sanctions (including fines and imprisonment) and/or civil sanctions (including civil penalties).

PS Form 3526, July 2014 (Page 3 of 3)

Moving?

Make sure your subscription moves with you!

To notify us of your new address, find your **Clinics Account Number** (located on your mailing label above your name), and contact customer service at:

Email: journalscustomerservice-usa@elsevier.com

800-654-2452 (subscribers in the U.S. & Canada)
314-447-8871 (subscribers outside of the U.S. & Canada)

Fax number: 314-447-8029

Elsevier Health Sciences Division
Subscription Customer Service
3251 Riverport Lane
Maryland Heights, MO 63043

Moving?

Make sure your subscription moves with you!

To notify us of your new address, find your **Clinics Account Number** (located on your mailing label above your name), and contact customer service at:

Email: journalscustomerservice-usa@elsevier.com

800-654-2452 (subscribers in the U.S. & Canada)
314-447-8871 (subscribers outside of the U.S. & Canada)

Fax number: 314-447-8029

Elsevier Health Sciences Division
Subscription Customer Service
3251 Riverport Lane
Maryland Heights, MO 63043

*To ensure uninterrupted delivery of your subscription, please notify us at least 4 weeks in advance of move.

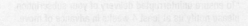